Hospice: the living idea

Edited by

Cicely Saunders DBE, MA, MD, FRCP, Hon DSc (Yale)
Medical Director, St Christopher's Hospice

Dorothy H. Summers SRN, RNT
Co-ordinator of Studies, St Christopher's Hospice

Neville Teller MA (Oxon)
Assistant Secretary, Department of Health and Social Security

D1211795

W. B. Saunders Company

© Cicely Saunders, Dorothy H. Summers and Neville Teller for St Christopher's, 1981

First published 1981
by Edward Arnold (Publishers) Ltd
41 Bedford Square, London WC1B 3DQ

Distributed in the United States by W. B. Saunders Company, West Washington Square, Philadelphia, PA 19105.

ISBN 0-7216-7931-5
Library of Congress Catalog Card Number 81-51725

Printed in Great Britain

Contributors

Ina Ajemian MD
Physician in Charge, Palliative Care Service,
Royal Victoria Hospital, Montreal, Canada

The Rev Canon John Austin Baker BLitt, MA(Oxon)
Canon of Westminster
Rector of St Margaret's Westminster
Chaplain to the Speaker of the House of Commons

Mary J. Baines MB BCh
Consultant Physician,
St Christopher's Hospice, London

Thelma D. Bates MB ChB FRCP MCRA
Consultant Radiotherapist and Oncologist,
St Thomas' Hospital, London SE1

Sister Zita Marie Cotter SCL
Family Nurse Practitioner, Las Vegas, USA

Loma Feigenberg MD
Associate Professor of Psychiatry (Thanatology)
Radiumhemmet, Karolinska Sjukhuset, Stockholm, Sweden

Robert Fulton PhD Sociology
Professor of Sociology, University of Minnesota,
Director, Center for Death Education and Research

Judith van Heerden MB ChB
Senior Medical Officer
Radiotherapy Department, Provincial Hospital
Port Elizabeth, South Africa

John Hinton MD DPM FRCP FRCPsych.
Professor of Psychiatry,
Middlesex Hospital Medical School, London

Rosemary Howarth RN
Sister-in-Charge
Oncology Unit, Royal Perth Hospital, Australia

Marilijn de Jong-Vekemans RN
Antonius Ijsselmonde Nursing Home, Rotterdam, Holland

Stephen R. Kirkham MRCP
Research Registrar,
St Christopher's Hospice, London

Samuel C. Klagsbrun MD
Medical Director, Four Winds Hospital, Katonah, USA

Janet Lunceford RN MSN
Project Officer, Hospice Program
Program Director for Oncology Nursing,
National Cancer Institute, Bethesda, USA

Ida M. Martinson, RN PhD FAAN
Professor of Nursing and Director of Research,
University of Minnesota School of Nursing,
Minneapolis, USA

Ronald Melzack PhD
Professor, Department of Psychology,
McGill University, Montreal, Canada

Balfour M. Mount MD FRCS(C)
Director, Palliative Care Service,
Professor, Department of Surgery,
Royal Victoria Hospital, Montreal, Canada

Greg Owen
Project Director, Terminal Care Study,
Amherst H Wilder Foundation, St Paul, Minnesota, USA

Dame Cicely Saunders DBE MA MD FRCP Hon DSc (Yale)
Medical Director, St Christopher's Hospice, London

John F. Scott MD MDiv
Director, Palliative Care Service,
St Michael's Hospital, Toronto, Canada

Mary Smith
Medical Secretary, St Christopher's Hospice, London

L. J. de Souza MS FRCS FRCSE FCPS
Assistant Surgeon, Tata Memorial Hospital,
Managing Trustee, Shanti Avedna Ashram, Bombay, India

Dorothy H. Summers SRN RNT
Co-ordinator of Studies, St Christopher's Hospice, London

Paul Torrens MD MPH
Professor of Health Services Administration,
University of California, Los Angeles, USA

T. D. Walsh MSc MRCP
Research Fellow, St Christopher's Hospice, London

Thomas S. West OBE MB BS
Deputy Medical Director,
St Christopher's Hospice, London

Eric Wilkes OBE MA FRCP FRCGP MRCPsych DObst RCOG
Professor of Community Care and General Practice,
Department of Community Medicine, University of Sheffield

Sir George Young, Bt MP
Parliamentary Under-Secretary of State (Health and Personal Social
Services), Department of Health and Social Security

Preface

'Like all good movements the impact of the hospice movement does not depend on bricks and mortar but on the interest its ideas generate and the changes in practical care which these have brought about.'

Sir George Young,
Parliamentary Under-Secretary of State,
Department of Health and Social Security

In June 1980, 68 people involved in various ways in hospice care came from 16 countries for a five-day conference at St Christopher's Hospice, joining workers in this field from the United Kingdom and members of St Christopher's staff. Two days were spent visiting other hospice units and teams and on the final day people from many other centres involved in what has become known as 'the hospice movement' came to hear reports of its world-wide and diverse development.

Hospice or palliative or continuing care aims to help those for whom the acute hospital is not appropriate and for whom the ordinary community services are no longer adequate. It is concerned with the quality of life remaining for them and for their families. Although its main concentration so far has been with those with advanced or terminal malignant disease, a few hospices have always welcomed some long-stay patients and the frail elderly.

The title Bar Mitzvah was chosen for the Conference as a reference to the Jewish patient who gave the founding gift and first ideas which led to the opening of St Christopher's Hospice in 1967. Past and present hospice practice was reviewed together with the analysis and research that are gradually establishing its scientific foundations. Challenges for the future, including the need for better evaluation and documentation, were presented.

The contributors were asked to speak to papers prepared for publication and most of these form this book. In order to keep it within reasonable compass two important papers were regretfully omitted as their subjects are well covered elsewhere; namely, the pharmacology of pain control (Twycross 1978, 1980) and a review of current geriatric practice, (Green 1978, 1980, 1981). That hospice care may be considered to be a facet of gerontology as it is of oncology, neurology and other disciplines was emphasized repeatedly at the conference as the participants looked at areas of need calling for future work.

It was obvious that the Conference believed that their work should be integrated with general medical practice, forming a complementary local resource and service. They recognized that much excellent 'hospice care' was carried out without use of the title and that the greatest impact of the movement may have already been on the way that people are being cared for in conventional settings.

This will develop further as those concerned in the movement accept the responsibilities of research and teaching, continually analysing, refining and evaluating their work. This book, in assessing the progress and practice of the last thirteen years and in looking to the future challenges of all kinds, is a step in this direction. The chapters that follow may strike the reader as unduly disparate, both in content and in style. Yet in a real sense these papers reflect the breadth of challenge of hospice work, which reconciles the discipline of applied science with the philosophy of personal care. The purpose behind the approach is by all the means at our command to enable patients and their families to find meaning in, and to use to the full, the time that remains to them.

Our grateful thanks go to the Tudor Trust and the Kaiser Family Foundation whose financial support made the Conference possible and to all the contributors and participants. I also thank my hard worked fellow editors, Dorothy Summers for all the organizing that went into the smooth running of the Conference and Neville Teller for his detailed labours with the manuscripts. Above all, our thanks go to the patients, families and staff who have shared their experiences with us.

1981
Sydenham   Cicely Saunders

References

Green, M. (1978). *Health in Middle Age,* Wayland, Hove, E. Sussex.

Green, M. (1980). When Widowhood Follows Retirement. In *Cruse Newsletter,* London.

Green, M. (1981). A Decade of the Advances in the Medicine of Old Age. *Geriatric Medicine.* **11,** 6.

Twycross, R. (1978). Relief of Pain. In *The Management of Terminal Disease,* Ed. by C. Saunders, Edward Arnold, London

Twycross, R. (1980). The Relief of Pain in Far-Advanced Cancer. *Regional Anesthesia.* **5,** 2.

Contents

1
The hospice concept

Hospice and health care

Sir George Young Bt MP

The hospice movement began here in Britain, spearheaded by the remarkable efforts of Dame Cicely Saunders, backed by her able and dedicated St Christopher's team. We are justifiably proud of the movement.

In this country the National Health Service is a comprehensive service designed to meet a wide range of needs, and many successful developments have been initiated by those working within it. It was partially built on a long and honourable tradition of voluntary effort: in 1948 the new NHS incorporated an excellent existing network of voluntary hospitals. Before that time most specialist services had been developed within those hospitals funded from charitable sources. The hospice movement has inherited this voluntary tradition, for even with a National Health Service there will always be room for independent groups to identify unmet needs and alternative ways of approaching problems. We are fortunate that in the thirty years of the NHS the statutory services have been continually enriched by the activities of charitable groups.

The pioneers of the hospice movement identified a very great need. This had not only been neglected by the conventional services but it was an area largely avoided by the public at large. The movement has been prepared to look death—the great taboo subject of our age—squarely in the face and to encourage the dying and their families and all those caring for them to do the same. It was recognized that only by facing the problems honestly could fear of death be relieved and the problems of the dying be overcome; that by controlling pain, relieving unpleasant symptoms and providing strong emotional support death could be natural and dignified instead of a daunting and dehumanizing process. Happily, there is now much more open discussion by the health care professions and the general public of the needs of the dying, but the initial achievement of the pioneers of terminal care in opening up the whole subject for examination, research and debate cannot be underestimated.

The hospice movement in this country is made up of groups which are largely independent. Their common aim has been to fill the gaps in existing services for the dying by establishing—and I stress the word—a *complementary* local service. This is undoubtedly the key to their success—apart, of course, from the very high quality care they have set out to provide. The pioneers of the movement made quite sure that their service 'was not isolated or separate from the traditional network of care and they have sought to forge close links with the NHS. A well-thought-out hospice scheme can considerably enhance overall health care provision in a particular locality, and health authorities have powers to make arrangements to contribute financially to the hospice's work. They may contract to support a specific number of beds or give an annual grant. An alternative approach was developed by the National Society for Cancer Relief which has raised the money to build and equip ten units in hospital grounds; it has then handed them over to the area health authority whose responsibility they have become. The Government warmly supports all the mechanisms which enable the voluntary sector and the NHS to co-operate closely. Because of such arrangements and because neither hospice nor NHS care is provided on a commercial basis, it is possible to achieve the maximum flexibility. It is possible to develop channels of communication which ease the transfer of an individual patient from hospital to home and from home to hospice and so ensure that he receives exactly the right sort of care at exactly the right time as his illness progresses.

A further advantage of the close involvement of hospices with the conventional services is that it has helped the hospice concept of care to become more widely known. The pioneers of the movement have never sought to retain a monopoly of their ideas. On the contrary, they have been keen to explain their philosophy and share their knowledge with those providing traditional forms of care. Like all good movements the impact of the hospice movement does not depend on bricks and mortar but on the interest its ideas generate and the changes in practical care which these have brought about.

To my mind this is where the real importance of the movement lies. There is still so much to be done to ensure that all dying patients receive sympathetic and comprehensive care, whether they die at home, in a hospital or in a hospice. There is a real need to improve the support that their families receive so that the desolation of bereavement can be alleviated as far as possible. The incidence of illness among newly bereaved widows and widowers increases markedly and it seems clear that improved bereavement support would be a useful preventive measure benefitting the whole health service as well as those families concerned.

The quickest way to ensure that the standard of terminal care is generally improved is to ensure that more staff receive information about the techniques of terminal care or have an opportunity to obtain further training or experience in them.

In this area the hospices are likely to become increasingly important in the future. They will have a developing role as centres of expertise and training. As always, St Christopher's is in the forefront here. My Department supports their unique Study Centre which provides training and information on terminal care for a wide range of health services' personnel. My Department also funds several Joint Board of Clinical Nursing Studies Courses on 'Care of the Dying' at other hospices. In the future I would like to see more hospices developing their own capacity to educate and inform so that eventually every region has access to at least one terminal care training resource.

A recent development which is doing a great deal to spread the word about good care for the dying has been the increasing interest in home care support teams. By working closely with the primary care team—general practitioners, district nurses and health visitors—such specialist teams can help raise standards of terminal care within the community. This is very important as so many people would like to die in their own homes if at all possible. Such teams started out as a natural and useful extension of the work of hospices. It is particularly good to see that many local voluntary groups have appreciated that while it takes time to raise the enormous sums involved in a capital project the terminally ill need support immediately. Therefore, they have started their efforts to improve care in their areas by funding one or two specialist nurses to work within the community. There is clearly scope for further exploration of the ways in which community support for the dying patient can be improved and extended and I believe that this will also be an important area in the future.

The hospice movement has developed techniques, such as those to control pain, which are relevant to other aspects of medicine. However, it can teach the health service in general about something more than terminal care or specific treatment techniques. By its very existence it offers a wider challenge to the health professions. It is pointing to factors which have perhaps been forgotten in the medical profession's quest for cures and the nursing profession's striving for technical excellence. It reminds staff that there is an additional dimension to their patients; that we should not be so busy developing curative medicine that we forget to care for people as individuals whose time in hospital is but a small part of their lives. Training and experience in terminal care can only enhance the general approach of professional staff, no matter where they work. But perhaps too, all those concerned with general basic training should look to the hospice movement and ask themselves what lessons are still to be learned about the way we approach patients and their families. It may be that those lessons should become an essential component in training so that they become a consistent thread running through the approach to all forms of patient care. The hospice movement seems to offer us a much needed antidote to a too heavy reliance on technological medicine. It certainly does not reject technology but it begs us to reassess its role in medicine and patient care.

The founding philosophy

Dame Cicely Saunders DBE

It is now thirty-two years since St Christopher's founding patient died. Yet David Tasma of Warsaw still has a place in our network of relationships and his words remain living and developing among us. I met him in my first ward as a social worker in St Thomas' Hospital way back in 1947, and I knew then the truth that he was dying, which he did not. So I followed him up and I waited, and when he was admitted to another hospital it was in fact I who finally told him. The foundation of St Christopher's is how we coped with that truth together. He needed skills which were not then available, but still more he needed a sense of belonging and somehow to find meaning. And as he remembered his grandfather, the Rabbi, he made peace with the God of his fathers. When he died he left a £500 founding gift 'to be a window in your home'—a symbol of all kinds of openness being interpreted now in so many fascinatingly different ways.

We moved out of the National Health Service, with a great deal of its interest and support, in order to build round that window. We moved out so that attitudes and knowledge could move back in and in working for that we have used so often another phrase of his which is also symbolic—'I want what is in your mind and in your heart'—setting out, I suppose, a dichotomy: truth of the mind in skill and understanding with truth of the heart in vulnerable friendship. David needed peace from distress to sort out who he was, to find how he could gather the scattered fragments of what looked an unfulfilled life somehow into a whole at its ending, to find meaning in having been and perhaps hope in going on being. In that phrase he sets us to look at the two meanings of the word philosophy. In the dictionary we find it refers to all the knowledge belonging to a particular branch of learning but that it also refers to the fundamentals that underlie branches of learning—ways of looking at things, how we do things but also why we do them. In the hospice movement we continue to be concerned both with the sophisticated science of our treatments and with the art of our caring, bringing competence alongside compassion.

That makes me think of other dichotomies. How does one balance a total focus on the needs of the individual with one's responsibility to the whole community? How does one hold together in a kind of creative tension the assurance of faith with the flexibility of tolerance? It is as if one were continually putting up two different poles and letting the sparks fly between. The truth is that we must preserve a readiness to ask new questions and seek new truth in all spheres. By establishing what look like opposites and not trying to achieve a false reconciliation, we may end by showing in fact that they can co-exist. A bar mitzvah is a good moment to do this.

Hospice—a developing role

Samuel C. Klagsbrun

There was a King a long time ago who had the sad misfortune of having a grown-up son who believed he was a turkey. The young man would sit under the table in the nude, pecking away at his food as a turkey might. The King was beside himself; he asked all the wise people in the world to come and advise him. 'How do I take care of my son? What do I do?' No one could help him.

Finally, an old, wise Rabbi was called, a wonderful, bearded old scholar. He came and looked at the young man. After a moment he got undressed, went under the table and joined him. The young man said 'What are you doing here?' and the Rabbi said 'I'm a turkey.'

'You're a turkey too?'

'Yes, I'm a turkey.'

So every day they both sat under the table and pecked away. Finally one day the Rabbi said 'You know what? Us turkeys, we get cold down here. I think we could still be turkeys and get dressed.' So he called for some clothes and they both got dressed and pecked away at the floor under the table.

A few days later the Rabbi said 'It's really kind of lonely down here. We could still be turkeys and eat at the table.' So gradually, still believing he was a turkey, the young man became a human being again.

In order to be effective in hospice care we believe we must understand the patient's spirit and know what it is like from the patient's point of view.

The year 1980 saw the coming of age of St Christopher's Hospice. It has been fun for thirteen years being fussed over while being impish and mischievous, upsetting the old guard and, by implication, telling everybody how terrible they all were. It has been a great, creative time of growth and development, but it has also been a time of mistakes. We found ourselves having to overcome childhood diseases which almost killed us. And whether it was the support of providence or good parents who came in and protected us periodically, we survived. We are now faced with sobering insights and greater expectations than ever before. We have reached the age of sexual procreation, spawning other hospices, who like all children, are often quite different from ourselves. We now have to assume new and greater adult responsibilities. What a shame! It is far less fun reaching the burdensome age of maturation. There is a less well-known tradition which takes place at the celebration of the bar mitzvah of a young person. Parents of a bar mitzvah quietly on the eve of the celebration turn to each other and say 'Baruch shepetarani', which in translation means 'Thank God we are rid of him!'.

Until the age of bar mitzvah the responsibility of a child rests squarely on the shoulders of the parents. At the age of bar mitzvah the parents bless the moment of shedding responsibility and transferring the entire burden, both good and bad, on to the shoulders of the child. As a bar mitzvah, St Christopher's and, by extension, the modern hospice movement are now totally responsible for themselves. They cannot hide behind ignorance, lack of knowledge or lack of experience. What then, are the responsibilities of the hospice movement for the future?

There is absolutely nothing in what has been achieved in the hospice movement which could not apply to the broadest aspects of health care. Hospice care is a misnomer when applied only to the dying patient and the issues surrounding death. The next thirteen years ought to focus on the expansion of the hospice concept with the aim of making all illness and its treatment the focus of attention of the hospice approach.

The hospice movement has an obligation to move towards three goals: the first is to refine and identify those aspects of hospice care which work. The ingredients of hospice care which have been most clearly publicized have been those based on pain management and qualities of home care. To be a bit cold blooded about it, the reason why pain management has been picked up around the world is not only because of its value, which is obvious, but also because of its technology. This is knowledge which can be documented, put into charts and translated into mechanical action rather easily. In an odd way, taking care of physical things seems to require a technique more than a person. As for the popularity of home care aspects of hospice, part of the reason is that home care is less expensive. It does not require an institution to make a commitment; all that is required is a cadre of volunteers under the leadership of a small number of committed people. It requires families' co-operation who, since they face the absence of any alternative method of care that is decent, seem to have very little choice in the matter. And so, to a degree, for hospice to be widely known because of pain management and home care concepts misses the point.

To refine and identify what hospice is all about means to focus on the people doing hospice care. The endless hours of spoon-feeding a patient at the bedside, the style of humour with which we approach a patient, the spiritual quality of commitment surrounding the patient, that is clearly what hospice care is about. How does one refine and identify those qualities? More important, how does one package and sell them? The best method is teaching, not by lecture and demonstration alone, but by example: teaching by doing and inviting other people to do the same. The proliferation in America of hospice courses and training programmes and the focus on techniques is a glaring example of misunderstanding of what hospice is all about.

Thus one task for the future is that of defining more clearly those qualities which make up a hospice. Sociologists might be asked to help describe the atmosphere that is the hospice; the qualities of interaction; the way hierarchy functions while remaining open to feelings. Associated with this will be the need to bring into much sharper focus the crucial and central importance of the spiritual dimension of working in a hospice. A hospice need not be a religious organization, but I do not exactly know how to conceptualize a hospice that can maintain itself and its philosophy and continue to have a sense of the meaningfulness of life in the midst of continual losses and visible suffering, without having recourse to a dimension beyond the individual and the self. That does not necessarily have to be a religious dimension but paying careful attention for the sake of the long-term survival of the hospice, if nothing else, to that spiritual dimension of its structure is a crucial and central factor of hospice life. To the rational human being suffering and death ultimately have to make sense in order for the person to remain human. I would hate to see a hospice staff develop a concentration camp survivor approach to life. Hospice care has now been in existence long enough to allow for research efforts on the impact of doing this kind of work on the staff. Is there need for concern for the quality of life of the staff? Does this work affect personal relationships? Does 'burn out' occur? Is there depression? Is there repressed anger? Answers to these and other issues may teach us about the steps necessary to improve the quality of life in hospice work not only for the patient but also for staff.

The second task for the future is the application of the hospice concept to a much broader segment of medicine. Obviously, geriatric care is an area which deserves attention from the hospice movement. Chronic diseases are a second area which clearly deserves that kind of focus. People whose lives have been constricted by an impairment of a significant kind deserve to be exposed to a hospice-like approach. The humanization of medicine in the face of ever-increasing technology is what the next thirteen years of hospice deserves and has a responsibility to influence.

Imagine an institution the job of which is to take care of old people with varying degrees of problems resulting from the ageing process, setting up a system which pays very careful and detailed attention to every small symptom, complaint or impairment of an old person. Imagine a pharmacologist or psychologist spending research time on all of these detailed complaints and coming up with an approach, either by virtue of medication or techniques aimed at ameliorating and minimizing some of them. Imagine a patient atmosphere where endless time is spent taking care of older people. In short, imagine a hospice devoted to the care of the elderly. What a revolution that would bring about in the treatment of the aged! Yet it would not be a truly technological revolution, but simply a change in attitude on the part of medical people towards segments of the population who are not found at present to be very exciting, challenging or interesting in the usual medical sense. By implication I am also talking about a change in medical care brought about by that shift in attitude of our colleagues in medicine. To me that is still, to this very day, the most frustrating part of hospice work.

If we are to be successful in having hospice concepts applied to medical areas beyond the terminally ill, we will have to find a better way to reach our colleagues. We ought to stop berating them for being insensitive, lacking in humanity, and for running away from emotions. Our job, frankly, is to find a more convincing way of reaching them. My sense is that we have to prove that we are providing a service which will benefit them as well as the patients and their families. We can, to some degree, take a burden off their hands and free them to do more of what they want to do. Our approach to date has been to invite physicians to see our work and learn to adapt our techniques to theirs. A more successful approach might be to develop teams of physicians, nurses and social workers to go out and relieve hospitals of the burden of having to take care of terminal patients by taking over responsibility for their care. Working in that fashion, our approach and our philosophy will blend into the institution by the process of osmosis, if not identification. The result of helping our colleagues may be that they end up doing more of what we want them to do.

Few of us have ended up working alongside primary care physicians, offering hospice care or aspects of hospice care to patients who are still undergoing active treatment. We have not sufficiently lent our voices to the improvement of patient care early enough. If it is true that preparation for terminal phases of life needs to take place at the time of active treatment, possibly even beginning with a diagnostic work-up, should there not be a place for hospice philosophy in an acute care hospital setting? If we want to expose all patients to hospice treatment, we will have to reach all physicians first.

The third responsibility for the hospice movement in the next thirteen years is to take heed of the incredible impact of a hospice environment on the mood of the patient and the family, and even on the occasionally changing behaviour of the continuing disease. We must explore the implication of how a good environment can cause a change in the attitude of the patient, and the potential of that change influencing the actual course of disease.

Hospice research over the next thirteen years must concentrate on exploring not only our emotional and spiritual impact on our patients but also what actually happens to the process of disease when our patients feel well taken care of, free of pain and are able to relate again. Longevity studies correlated with change in attitudes must be undertaken. As an extension of such studies, implications of good management, change in attitudes of patients as well as families and change in atmosphere caused by hospice care must be studied, together with the long-term effects of that experience on the subsequent life patterns of families and staff going through such an experience. Does this care matter beyond the immediate moment in life when it is rendered? Does an offspring deal with stress as a future adult differently because of this unique experience? How often do people remarry, divorce, have other children in the hospice-treated population as opposed to families not exposed to hospice care? These and many other questions need major attention.

The care of the dying is the care of all of us. What we learn from the dying applies to all of us during life. In a way it is the dying who are giving us a much better awareness of the gift of life. It is they who are our best teachers.

Hospice in America

From principle to practice*

Robert Fulton and Greg Owen

Current efforts to provide compassionate care for the dying, which today is embodied in the concept of hospice, has a long and honourable history in which all nations and peoples have played a part.

Consider, for example, the bravery and mercy of St Bridget in Ireland during the fifth century, a time marked by brutal atrocities, savage warfare and pagan worship, or that of Brother Gerard and the Hospitaller Knights of St John and their selfless courage at the time of the crusades. Brother Vincent de Paul and his Sisters of Charity in Paris are to be remembered too, as is the work of Reverend Fleidner at Kaiserwerth Hospital in Prussia. Another link in the chain was Father Damien's work among the lepers of Molowkai; then there was the Quaker, Elizabeth Fry, and her efforts on behalf of patients and their families in England, and Sister Mary Aikenhead who founded the Irish Sisters of Charity in Dublin in 1815 which ultimately led to the establishment of St Joseph's Hospice in Hackney in 1905.

The founding of St Christopher's in Sydenham in 1967 could be said to be the final step in the synthesis of the modern form of hospice care; but at the same time it could be described as the first step in providing a compassionate witness to the dying for the world community. Wherever one may look, therefore, whatever spiritual mandate one might examine, the impulse to provide care, comfort and relief to persons in need, ill or confronted by death is as ancient and universal as it is inspiring. In the western world, such a calling may be traced to the Parable of the Good Samaritan, the seven acts of mercy and, ultimately, the love of Christ.

A discussion of American hospice development properly begins with a description of Hospice, Inc. of New Haven, Connecticut. This programme began at Yale University where Dr Cicely Saunders first spoke to American audiences in 1963. Florence Wald, Edward Dobihal, Ira Goldenberg, Morris Wessel and Kathryn Klaus prepared and completed an *Interdisciplinary Study for Care of Dying Patients and Their Families* in 1969, and organized a steering committee in the spring of 1971 to consider the development of a hospice programme in the New Haven area. The group was incorporated later that same year, just four years after the opening of St Christopher's in London. Hospice, Inc. began home care service in 1974

*The authors wish to thank the Northwest Area Foundation and the Amherst H Wilder Foundation, both of St Paul, Minnesota, for their generous support of this project. We also extend our appreciation to Dr David Berger and Dr Paul Mattessich for their assistance in the design and implementation of the study upon which this report is based.

and has recently dedicated a newly designed facility in Branford, Connecticut.

The national leadership of Hospice, Inc. in the area of hospice programme development in the United States can be seen in their service as a clearing house for hospice information in the United States, their co-ordination and sponsorship of National Symposia on Hospice Care, their contractual arrangements with the then Department of Health, Education and Welfare and the National Cancer Institute in studying the provision and utilization of hospice services, their active dialogue with state and federal officials on the need to licence and accredit hospice programmes, their development of national standards for hospice care and their successful application to the US Patent and Trade Mark Office for ownership of the term 'hospice' as a nationally registered service mark. This was awarded to Hospice, Inc. in 1978 and ownership has since been transferred to the National Hospice Organization (NHO), a non-profit organization incorporated in Washington, DC. The leadership of the NHO, established at the Second National Hospice Symposium in 1977, is composed of hospice programme developers from various parts of the United States.

We believe that it is correct to say that the initial responsiveness of American audiences to the hospice message of compassionate care and the relief of pain was conditioned in great part by the work of Dr Elisabeth Kubler-Ross and particularly by her book, *On Death and Dying*, which exposed a sensitive nerve in the health care delivery system of the United States. This widely read book crystallized for the hospital nurse in particular the problems faced by those whose task it was to deal with the private issues of death in a public setting. In short, what Dr Ross said was that we must attend to the death of another with our hearts as well as with our minds. The death of a fellow human being could not take place ignominiously in the obscurity of back wards and darkened rooms without such deaths casting dark shadows across the lives of us all.

Her important and timely message to nurses and other care-givers across the country touched their hearts as it reached the public's ears and the effect was electrifying. Moreover, her book appeared at the time when the outraged reaction of Americans toward the Vietnam War was at its zenith and when the cold, mechanistic attitude of the Administration toward the war and its victims was being publicly scrutinized. The Government's denigration of life and depersonalization of death as reported in the daily news did much to galvanize public sentiment and lift up private emotions.

It is important to note, too, that at the time Dr Saunders came to the United States there was an alternative proposal being vigorously advocated in the form of the euthanasia movement. Responding to the loneliness, isolation, lack of family involvement and unrelieved pain that came to be synonymous with individuals dying in acute care hospitals, concerned persons in the euthanasia movement advocated the right to die either by assisting the patient to end his or her life, or by the discontinuance of treatment. Robert Veatch of the Hastings Center reported in 1977 that forty pieces of legislation were introduced into state legislatures during this period in an attempt to legalize one or another aspect of euthanasia.

The effect of the hospice movement on these different efforts is not to be underestimated. Hospice proponents have emphasized the quality of remaining life and the ability of attending care-givers to provide comfort and care rather than an extreme solution to the problem of patient distress. The hospice philosophy, in confronting the euthanasia movement head on, has not only illuminated the problems of dying as never before, but has also provided a more humane and acceptable manner of dealing with these problems. The success and acceptance of the hospice movement by professional care-givers and family members alike can be measured by the fact that the Euthanasia Educational Council has recently seen fit to change its name to Concern for Dying as an expression, in part, of their support and belief in the principles of the hospice movement.

In the past six years, since the founding of the New Haven Hospice, we have seen the number of hospice programmes in the United States increase to well over 200, with virtually every small and large city now involved in some kind of hospice planning. This is no accident, it is no fad and it is no temporary enthusiasm. Major insurance companies including Blue Cross and Blue Shield and American Family, as well as Federal health care reimbursement programmes such as Medicare and Medicaid, are now providing some kind of hospice benefits and are exploring ways to expand their coverage. Major newspaper columnists such as Sylvia Porter have addressed the issue in week-long series of articles. All of the major news magazines and television networks have covered various aspects of the rapid developments in hospice care. Additionally, the number of books and articles on hospice care now exceeds 1000, where there existed virtually a handful only a decade ago. Finally, testimony to the worldwide response to the needs of those in distress and the preservation of our humanity is reflected in the award of the 1979 Nobel Peace Prize to a Catholic nun, Mother Teresa, who has devoted herself to the care of the dying in Calcutta.

In a world in which technology threatens to undermine our sense of worth and meaning, hospice has appeared with the promise of not only easing the course for those who must die, but also of restoring the fundamental familial and religious ideals that have nourished our civilization.

The current interest and concern for the dying that are evidenced by the burgeoning hospice movement in the United States cannot be explained, however, simply in terms of the evidence cited above. The American psyche has not suddenly embraced what it formerly denied. As Samuel Vaisrub, the editor of the *Journal of the American Medical Association*, reminded his readers recently, 'Death and dying have always been with us'. Indeed, academic interest in the subject began even prior to Thomas Eliot's work in the 1930s and has progressed almost uninterrupted ever since. This can be seen in the writings of Scott, Hall, Eissler, Feifel, Strauss, Sudnow, Fulton and others, to say nothing of numerous anthropological studies or the intermittent forays against American mortuary practices, such as Jessica Mitford's *The American Way of Death*, or Evelyn Waugh's *The Loved One*.

The singular interest in hospice, to say nothing of the ever-growing literature on death and dying, is attributable, we believe, to a convergence of different social and cultural factors. Prominent among these are the rise of secularism and the halting decline in traditional religious beliefs. Moreover, the general increase in life expectancy, the rapidly growing elderly population, the physical and social mobility of the American public, the de-ritualization of death and mourning, and the general insulation of young persons from the event of death have served to bring us to this present condition. The effect of these recent trends has been to segregate the aged, the chronically ill and the dying from the rest of the community and simultaneously to isolate the young from any direct experience with dying or death, the consequence of which is to rob both child and adult of these significant human relationships and experiences.

The de-ritualization of death and the suppression of grief and mourning that can be observed in contemporary society also serve to aggravate the isolation of the generations. Geoffrey Gorer, the distinguished English anthropologist, believes that such repudiation and denial of grief goes far to explain the rising tide of vandalism and violence that is presently reported among the young. More colourfully, Dr Richard Lamerton of St Joseph's Hospice, in a recent speech in America, characterized our present condition as 'the bottom of the trough, the running down of our civilization, and a time of ignorance and darkness'. In observing that hospice could perhaps be the beginning of a renaissance, and a much needed corrective for our troubled times, he expresses both the moral reaction and the creative humane response that hospice has come to represent.

In order to discuss the rapid proliferation of hospice programmes in the United States without reiterating what has already been said more completely by others, or what is already well known, permit us to describe the research that we have undertaken in the metropolitan region of Minneapolis and St Paul, Minnesota. We believe that the wide range of hospice programmes that have developed in this area, the issues that have emerged, the conflicts that have arisen and the successes that have been achieved allow us to say with confidence that what we have observed here in microcosm finds its counterpart throughout the entire country. We feel justified, therefore, in speaking broadly about the issues associated with the rise and development of hospices throughout the United States because of the intensive and extensive characer of local hospice activity. For example, the existing programmes found in the Twin City area represent a wide range of alternative methods for implementing hospice care, including separate wings in hospitals, home-care programmes, hospice teams serving throughout hospitals and programmes designed around oncology units. Moreover, the area is rich in national hospice leadership including Dr Robert Brown, the President-elect of the National Hospice Organization,

Carmian Seifert, the Chairperson of the Standards and Accreditation Committee of the NHO, and several hospice personnel who have gained direct experience in the Yale–New Haven environment.

All of these elements provide an excellent setting for assessing community sentiment toward hospice care and programmatic developments in hospice services. The presence of a free terminal cancer home administered by the Sisters of the Hawthorne Dominican Order adds further richness and historical balance to the work we have been able to do. Coupled with our correspondence and consultantships with outstate hospice programmes, we were able to study in detail the various issues facing hospice programmes and the personnel who serve them. The diverse nature of the thirteen Twin City programmes comprised of Protestant, Catholic and Jewish hospices as well as those without a religious affiliation, served as the basis for the study.

In the course of our study we had the opportunity to interview all but one of the local hospice directors, to interview a representative sample of 150 bereaved survivors, to sample by mail the opinions of nearly 150 local physicians as well as to survey the attitudes of 100 participating care-givers representing a variety of skills and services.

An important issue now being raised by health-care providers locally and throughout the country has to do with the degree of overlap between various health service programmes that are now operating and the growing number of hospices that wish to provide the complete set of hospice benefits. Home nursing services, housekeeping assistance, bereavement counselling, health education, as well as medical supplies for the home are now available in most large communities through a wide variety of service programmes, all of which have preceded the development of hospice. The existing programmes, moreover, are designed for use by a wider population of clients than those now served by hospice.

Concern is expressed by the persons providing these health services that the implementation of hospice programmes operating autonomously and independently might result in the needless duplication of effort while at the same time undermining the efforts of existing service providers. This was clearly expressed in the care-giver questionnaires. For example, one respondent stated:

> I wholeheartedly support the hospice concept as a humane approach to caring for terminally ill patients and their families. However, 'reality' issues such as cost-effectiveness, licence accreditation, *coordination of existing resources*, and community needs assessment are all issues that hospice providers must address.

Or again, another respondent wrote:

> Hospice, as it is developing, is eroding the legitimate, supportive care available to families through other programmes and giving the public the impression that they are deprived if they have been denied this prescription of care!
>
> This impression is demeaning to other caring health professionals who have dealt with terminal illness quite comfortably before the advent of this current programme of care.

The commitment of the National Hospice Organization to autonomous hospice administrations, with an emphasis on free-standing facilities and reimbursement procedures separate from existing health care coverage, stands in conflict with the goals of many local hospice directors who have expressed their desire to integrate hospice services within hospital programmes and to enhance thereby the quality of care offered to all persons regardless of diagnosis or prognosis. Additionally, such a position, it is contended, tends to undermine the morale of home health care providers who have been offering home care to dying persons for more than twenty years and who have now begun to incorporate advanced methods of pain and symptom relief, 24-hour service availability, and bereavement follow-up into their programmes. Clearly, hospice, as defined by the American NHO, will have an uphill battle with currently existing programmes for the dying that have preceded hospice and will increasingly receive pressure to co-operate with existing health care providers. Moreover, some rural hospice planning groups that have been forthright in their desire to keep their programmes simple and co-operative now stand in belligerent opposition to the NHO, which is perceived as attempting to monopolize the field through their particular definition of hospice without regard for the needs of rural areas. Their antagonism is further fired by the fact that the NHO now owns the term 'hospice' as a nationally registered service mark and is only willing to bestow the use of this term upon hospice programmes meeting or attempting to meet the national specifications. To what degree the NHO is willing to compromise in its expectations is as yet unknown, but there is no question that lines are now being drawn between the many hospital hospice programmes that have developed and the leadership of the National Hospice Organization.

In the Minneapolis and St Paul area, the problems inherent in rigidly defining hospice care are already visible. The desire on the part of concerned care-givers to offer hospice services to their dying patients has resulted in a variety of 'patchwork' programmes.

But two beds on a medical-surgical unit with some in-service death education, combined with a home care nurse and a liberalized policy of pain relief does not constitute a bonafide hospice programme in the minds of NHO proponents. For example, our survey has found that some physicians choose to refer patients to hospices for home care services only. When the need for in-patient care arises, the patient is then admitted to another hospital, typically the one in which the physician has medical privileges; out-patient care in such cases is handled from the physician's office.

Other physicians, while expressing support for the hospice concept, are reluctant, nevertheless, to see yet another new programme established. They feel that continuity of patient care would be better served by a greater utilization and co-ordination of existing programmes. This is, in fact, the way in which most of the local hospice programmes are conceived and organized. Individuals with nursing or seminary backgrounds have been hired as hospice co-ordinators and are expected to bring the full scope of the hospital's resources to bear on the needs of their terminally ill patients. These co-ordinators, moreover, are increasingly becoming involved in oncology care for purposes of educating and supporting the patient and family immediately following diagnosis. Consequently, the hospice concept is being projected and extended to new areas of health care service even as it is being formally defined by the National Hospice Organization.

Thus, the desire on the part of the NHO to prescribe the total programme of care that for the most part conforms to the New Haven (Branford) model inevitably leads toward conflict with these and other local service providers who have no intention of sacrificing their programmes for the sake of national conformity. The fact that the NHO now owns the term 'hospice' as a national service mark means that those programmes that wish to be described as 'hospices' and receive NHO accreditation in the 1980s will have to conform to the national guidelines or contest the registration of 'hospice' as a privately owned service mark.

The local ramifications of this problem were apparent at a recent meeting of the Hospice Collaboration Committee of the Minnesota Coalition for Terminal Care. It was decided that the newly formed Minnesota Hospice Organization would include as voting members only those providers who would eventually comply with NHO guidelines. Some hospice providers felt abandoned by this decision and no longer participate in the meetings. What is promised by this development is a split between metropolitan hospitals that have the resources to provide the full scope of hospice services and rural and surburban hospitals that do not.

This controversy can be seen to extend into the area of reimbursement where the question of quality health care is constantly being weighed against the cost of providing such care. In contrast to the experience in Britain where a substantial proportion of beds is financed by the National Health Service, the American scene demonstrates a wide variety of third-party payment sources, all of which demand an accounting of health care dollars. Services such as co-ordination of care, physician home visits, supportive services of various types, homemaker assistance, bereavement support, as well as spiritual counselling, are not currently reimbursed under conventional health insurance programmes. Yet, such services constitute a significant dimension of the total hospice programme. Moreover, not only is the request being made for reimbursement of the proffered services but, given the staffing philosophy and practices of many American hospice programmes, a significant proportion of these services is now and later will be provided by non-credentialed personnel. Traditional mechanisms channel third-party payments primarily to physicians, acute care hospitals and nursing homes. Given the all-embracing objectives of hospice care, adequate financial support at this juncture is still a highly problematical issue. While studies such as the one conducted by our friend and colleague Dr Ida Martinson of Minnesota tend to suggest that large cost savings can be realized by emphasizing home care, other studies suggest that cost and savings tend to balance each other out given the demand that hospices make for more personnel, higher nurse : patient ratios and increased co-ordinative and supportive services.

At the moment, the issue of reimbursement is still very much in doubt and there will probably be no substantial changes in Federal policies and practices until the twenty-six hospices presently being funded by the Health Care Financing Administration have been completely evaluated.

Paradoxically, the issue of reimbursement as it affects the future course of the hospice movement in America may hinge upon the role of the volunteer. Yet, it can be said that it was the volunteer who established hospice. If reimbursement ultimately depends upon a credentialed care-giver, it might be expected that the future personnel structure of hospice programmes throughout the country will change radically.

But apart from this issue, there are still other forces at work that make the role of the volunteer in the service of hospice increasingly difficult. A powerful and vocal force in America today is the women's movement. Increasingly, women have become uncomfortable providing volunteer labour alongside other women who are compensated for their efforts. These are times, moreover, in which women as wives and mothers must cope with inflation and recession simultaneously. As a result, it becomes more difficult for the potential wage earner to provide free services in the face of personal need.

The attrition of volunteers can come from another quarter, however—from stress and one's inability ultimately to sustain oneself in the face of dying and death. That the volunteer is confronted with what is unfortunately described in the American literature as 'burnout'—no less so than their professional counterparts—has been frequently observed. It has also been observed that volunteers in hospice are particularly attracted to this work following recent bereavements of their own. The work of Dr Mary Vachon and her colleagues of the Clarke Institute at the University of Toronto have shown to what extent stress intrudes upon the ministrations of care-givers. That this is a problem in America to a degree possibly unknown elsewhere is due in part to the secular character of American society and the variety of hospice programmes it now supports. In contrast to St Christopher's, which is not only structurally autonomous but also maintains continuity of personnel, daily religious services, a variety of patient and staff programmes and such singular activities as the choir and Pilgrim's Club, the average American hospice programme is devoid of these culturally enriching activities and the profound religious underpinning that sustains the spirit of the care-giver. It is not surprising, therefore, to find that American hospice directors have turned to the mental health facilitator, the staff psychiatrist, self-help groups and various relaxation techniques for assistance in the absence of traditional support mechanisms and symbolic reinforcement of their emotionally burdened personnel.

Finally, there is the issue of the role of hospice within the larger medical care system in America. The high quality and intensity of care being provided in some hospice programmes has caused care-givers in other settings to wonder why their patients don't deserve the same high quality of care. In fact, one non-hospice patient jokingly enquired of his physician, 'Do you have to die to get that kind of care?' The point is not taken lightly by some care-givers, as was demonstrated at a recent regional medical conference held in St Paul, Minnesota. A woman at the conference expressed concern that the substantial resources being heaped upon a Veteran's Administration three-year pilot hospice programme in California could be equally well spent on many of the acute and chronically ill patients who are provided with far fewer hours of nursing care. She felt that all patients could benefit from the kind of compassionate attention that hospice promotes and suggested that the ideal outcome would be for hospices to 'self-destruct' after the hospice philosophy had been embodied throughout the health care system. What must be recognized by her remarks is that hospice has the potential to revolutionize the American health care system from the inside out. The prospect that hospice philosophy can bring about a 'revolution' in health care institutions is given support by the fact that various non-hospice programmes have already begun to incorporate hospice principles into their daily routines.

The acceptance of the hospice philosophy in America is a tangible recognition of the vitality of the values and principles that hospice care represents. Paradoxically, however, to the extent to which these principles are diffused throughout the entire health care system, one can observe increased resistance to the establishment of autonomous and separate hospice programmes.

In the final analysis, however, whatever the outcomes may be with respect to the several issues we have raised, it must be recognized that hospice constitutes a new social movement in America. It is a movement that reaches beyond itself as it challenges care-givers to extend themselves in service to others. To the degree that we as care-givers become involved personally and charitably in the lives of dying patients, rather than leaving such tasks to others, we find ourselves in new relationships with strangers in need. Hospice thus brings us to a post-Samaritan age—an age in which love and altruism, indeed, social life itself, are regenerated in the act of caring for those who suffer and die.

Authors' note

The text of this paper contains several references to the National Hospice Organization (NHO) that are now inaccurate. The inaccuracies are the result of the authors' reliance on materials published by the NHO prior to 1979. During the period 1979–1980, the aims and directions of the NHO changed dramatically, although these changes were not widely publicized, nor were they recognized by hospice providers in the study area.

Consequently, respondent's perceptions of the NHO and its activities are based primarily on materials distributed by the NHO prior to 1979. Concerning this information, the following points should be noted.

1. The NHO has now withdrawn its application to the US Patent and Trademark office for ownership of the term 'hospice' as a nationally registered service mark. (Materials published by the NHO in 1978 indicate that this service mark was awarded to Hospice, Inc. on February 14, 1978 with ownership to be transferred to the NHO.)

2. The NHO is no longer committed to: (a) autonomous hospice administrations; (b) the promotion of free-standing facilities; or (c) reimbursement mechanisms separate from existing coverage.

3. The NHO now publically endorses alternative ways of providing hospice services and wishes to co-operate with existing service providers in meeting NHO standards of care.

2
Hospice as a style for living

The adult patient: Cultural considerations in palliative care

Ina Ajemian and Balfour M. Mount

Introduction

The Palliative Care Service was instituted at the Royal Victoria Hospital, a 1000-bed teaching hospital affiliated with McGill University, in January 1975, in an attempt to meet better the total needs (physical, psychological, social and spiritual) of terminally ill patients and their families. The service comprises five clinical arms: an in-patient ward (the palliative care unit), a hospital-based home care programme, an out-patient clinic, a consultation service to the remainder of the hospital and a bereavement follow-up service. The Palliative Care Service (PCS) is staffed by a multidisciplinary team which includes physicians, nurses, volunteers, social worker, chaplain, physiotherapist, music therapist, psychiatrist, as well as education, research and administrative staff.

The first goal in treating patients where cure or prolongation of life are no longer attainable goals, is to ensure that they receive optimal symptomatic management. When pain and other symptoms are controlled or minimized, the multidisciplinary team can then turn its attention to the myriad psychological, social and spiritual concerns of the patient and family.

Each person—health professional, volunteer, patient or family member—has a unique understanding of life and its meaning. This has been moulded by ethnic origins, social class and family expectations, as well as previous exposure to religion and philosophy. The term 'culture' in social psychology, identifies the totality of one's symbolic heritage—one's way of living. When faced with crisis, particularly the ultimate crisis of impending death, we seek to understand our human predicament, to put our lives, our suffering, our experience, in some framework of meaning.

To be effective, members of the helping professions must first understand themselves in relation to their own social mores, prejudices, and world view—working out their own structure of meaning. Then, in meeting patients, they may be better able to see their patients' social context in perspective. If we fail to make these distinctions, we risk assessing our patients on the basis of our biases and labelling as psychopathology behaviour that is quite appropriate in the context of the patient.

It follows that we have least difficulty understanding the social and cultural context of a patient who shares our own ethnic background, language, culture of origin and religion or world view. Zborowski (1952) and Kalish and Reynolds (1976) have looked at various aspects of behaviour in relation to pain and death in a variety of ethno-cultural groups in the United States. No one has yet done similar studies in Canada.

Greater Montreal, from which Victoria Hospital draws its patients, is a large metropolitan city of enormous diversity, including large francophone and anglophone subgroups and minority groups representing first generation immigrants from around the world. This review looks at the following factors:

1. The profile of our patient population, compared to that of our staff.
2. Problems arising when there are significant social/cultural differences between staff and patients.
3. Approaches to bridging these differences so that we may provide better care for our patients.

Profile of patient population compared to that of staff

Method

Demographic data were collected on all 135 patients cared for on the Palliative Care Unit and Home Care Program during a six-month period. These were compared with data describing our professional and volunteer staff during the same period of time.

Results

1. Sex (Table 2.1).

Table 2.1

	Male (%)	Female (%)
Patients	42	58
Professional staff	24	76
Volunteers	15	85

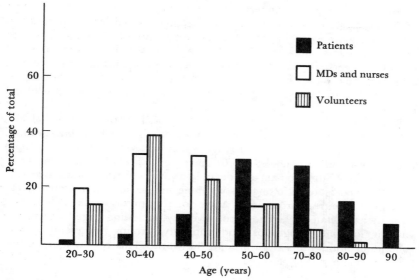

Fig. 2.1

2. Age (Fig. 2.1).
3. Marital status (Table 2.2).

Table 2.2

	Patients (%)	Staff (%)
Never married	9.6	26.5
Married	58.5	62.0
Separated or divorced	7.4	7.5
Widow(er)	24.4	4.0

4. Country of origin (Fig. 2.2).
5. Primary language (Fig. 2.3).
6. Patients with difficulty communicating because of language (Table 2.3).
7. Religion. In this category patients were asked their religious affiliations. No effort was made to establish how important personal faith was to a particular patient (Fig. 2.4).

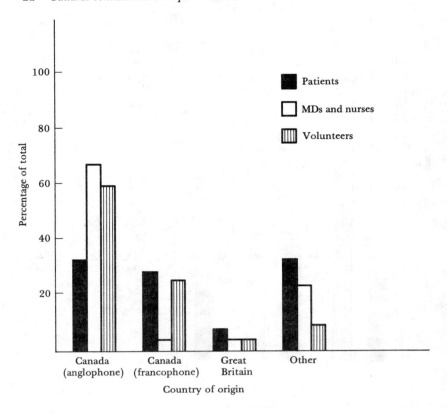

Fig. 2.2

Table 2.3

	Patients (%)
Difficulty in English	
None	55
Moderate	27
Extreme	18
Primary language of those having difficulty	
Francophone	23
Other	22

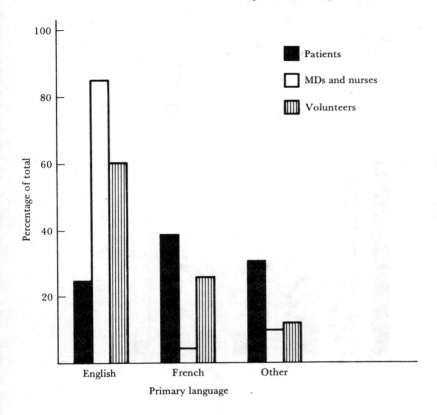

Fig. 2.3

Discussion

Medical teams have tended to be predominantly female because of the traditional female nurse role. In our staff, the female to male ratio was 3 : 1, while in the patient group the ratio was 3 : 2. It is worth remembering that some patients related more freely and easily with one or the other sex. If the professional team is predominantly female, male volunteers can be recruited to provide some balance.

Medical teams are composed primarily of young adults. The incidence of terminal illness related to malignant disease rises with advancing age. In our sample, 86 per cent of our staff were less than 50 years of age, while 86 per cent of the patient group were 50 years or more. Faced with impending death, patients may wish to reflect on their total life experience in evaluating the meaning of life. For an older patient, the sharing of these

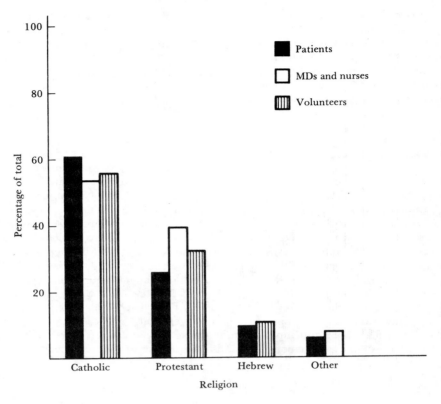

Fig. 2.4

thoughts will be modified if the care given is by a young person who has never experienced the social climate of decades past. For example, a nurse found it impossible to understand why a patient with limited life expectancy and serious material needs refused to use the life savings which he had kept 'for a rainy day'. She had never known the Depression of the '30s, nor the trauma of World War II. Balance in the team may again be improved by recruiting volunteers from all age groups.

A husband or wife facing the loss of a spouse, or parent facing the loss of a child, may not believe that a young unmarried staff person who has never known such a relationship can truly understand the depth of feeling such a loss involves. In our sample, 26 per cent of the staff have never been married. Only 4 per cent of the staff had lost a marriage partner by death. By comparison, only 10 per cent of the patient group had never married, and 24 per cent of the patient group had already experienced the death of a spouse. Widow–widow support groups, and groups of parents who have lost children, have demonstrated that often someone who has experienced a similar loss is particularly equipped to understand and be helpful. Again, this is a factor to consider in selecting volunteers who may add balance to the professional team.

Canada was the country of origin for 70 per cent of the staff and 86 per cent of the volunteers. By comparison, 41 per cent of the patient population came from countries outside Canada. On examining further the origin of this group, we find almost every European country represented as well as countries in the Middle and Far East. This implies an extremely wide range of social customs and expectations.

The language barrier present in communicating with many PCS patients was found to be significant. Patients were classified as having no difficulty, moderate, or extreme difficulty with spoken English. Those with 'moderate difficulty' were defined as having sufficient fluency to communicate basic daily needs, without the capacity to distinguish shades of meaning or emotions. The communication of emotionally charged material can be extremely difficult even in one's primary language. Attempts to express subtle feelings in a second language are even more problematic. Feelings are then frequently left unexpressed or stated indirectly using symbolic language. The greater the language barrier, the more impossible is adequate communication. Forty-five per cent of patients had moderate or extreme difficulty in English. Since most of the staff are French–English bilingual, communication with the primarily French-speaking patients was generally adequate. In our sample, however, fully 22 per cent of the patients had major difficulties communicating in both English and French. Since we define as a major goal ministering to the patients' psychosocial and spiritual needs, this presents an enormous challenge.

The religious orientations of our patient population, as defined by denominational affiliation, are quite similar to those of our staff and volunteers. Not indicated in this survey is the variation in tradition and expression within a denomination in different geographical locations. For example, one has only to look at the rapid evolution of the Roman Catholic Church in Canada in the past two decades to recognize that the religious experience and expectations of the foreign-born patient may be very different from those of the care-giver of the same faith.

Case reports

Case 1

A 66-year old Muslim man from Pakistan, speaking only Urdu, was admitted to the unit for control of incapacitating pain secondary to carcinoma of the prostate. During the admission, his wife was admitted to another hospital and subsequently died from a cerebrovascular accident. With analgesics, the patient was able to move more easily, but his face still looked haunted. Unable to share verbally, the staff attempted to communicate care and concern by touching his arm or shoulder. This upset him further. In an effort to relieve some of his distress, the patient was offered a tape recorder and selected tapes of music from India and Pakistan. He was very unhappy. Later, through an interpreter, he told us, 'In my religion music has no place, for it stands between me and my God—all I want to do now that I'm sick is pray to my God.' It also became clear that touching, particularly by female staff and volunteers, constituted, from his perspective, an inappropriate advance and an invasion of his privacy. One day a volunteer arrived who had spent her childhood in India and learned Urdu in school. She spoke to him in his language. His face lit up and, thereafter, whenever she was present the agony of his isolation was lifted.

Comment

As a Muslim, this patient was a follower of Islam, a word meaning, 'surrender', 'submission' or 'commitment into the hands of a sovereign divine ruler', a ruler whose will is to be followed in every aspect of life. The Muslim believes that nothing should be allowed to intervene in this relationship between man and his omnipresent God. Islam is a religion of law. Guidelines cover dress, social interaction, dietary customs and every other aspect of life (Parrinder, 1971). There are, for example, strict Muslim laws governing death-related rituals. The body is placed with the head toward Mecca. Ritual prayers said by those in attendance proclaim, 'all glory to Him who controls all things; unto Him you shall return.' The body is washed by relatives of the same sex as the patient and wrapped in pieces of cloth for immediate burial. Cement graves or coffins are not permitted. Respect for the body prevails, so no part of the body may be removed. *Post-mortem* examination and cremation are not allowed (Mufti Abdul Baqui).

In this instance, unable to communicate verbally and unfamiliar with the social and religious context of the patient, the staff attempted to communicate non-verbally, using physical contact and music. Both were inappropriate and added to the patient's discomfort.

Case 2

Mr G., a 79-year-old Jewish patient, was first visited in consultation and later transferred to the Palliative Care Unit, where he died two days later. His wife was with him constantly and was extremely sad and tearful. She spoke English well, but was grateful to have a volunteer speak to her in Yiddish, her first language. She expressed utter hopelessness at the prospect of life without her husband and said she had saved a number of sleeping pills to take as her solution when she could cope no longer. She believed there was a tradition that God would take good men on a Jewish high holy day. Yom Kippur occurred while he was on the PCU. When he was so very ill and yet did not die on that day she was confused; uncertain whether God was saving her husband for her, or judging her because she had not fasted for the holy day as her tradition prescribed. She questioned whether if she had had a stronger faith she would be better prepared to handle not only her present crisis but past losses throughout a difficult life. Her identity had always been intensely Jewish but in a cultural, rather than a religious sense.

During conversations with the staff, Mrs G. related details of the many losses she had experienced in her lifetime. When she was very young her father and brother were killed in Poland. During World War II, the patient and her husband were forced to move into a Ghetto and three days later their only daughter, aged 18, was taken by the Gestapo and never heard of again. They never ceased grieving for her. Later, Mrs G. and her husband escaped from the Ghetto and were hidden in an underground cave by Christian friends. After liberation, they relocated in Italy, then Israel, then Canada. Throughout their many trials, Mrs G. lived for and through her husband. After his death, Mrs G. felt lost and totally unable to venture outside the home without direction from others.

Comment

This lady's agony could not have been understood, except in the context of the psychological trauma she had suffered in the multiple losses of her life, particularly the unresolved grief for her daughter. Although the traumatic events of the Holocaust occurred more than thirty years ago, the effects persist in survivors, who often show decreased ability to tolerate subsequent life stresses (Chodoff, 1970; Hirschfeld, 1977). Frequently, no other family members survived and few subsequent interpersonal relationships have been established, resulting in profound guilt, loneliness, chronic depression and insomnia (Chodoff, 1970). Similar emotional disturbances have been noted in the children of survivors, even when born years after the Holocaust (Newman, 1979).

When a lifetime of recurrent pain precedes the current crisis, coping patterns, adaptive or maladaptive, are deeply ingrained and realistic goals should focus on support for the current event rather than more intensive therapy. Hirschfeld (1977) gives some useful guidelines for nursing interventions with such patients, including the following.

1. Work toward establishing basic trust, aware that there may be severe impairment of the survivor's ability to form or accept interpersonal relationships.

2. Set realistic goals based on an assessment of available psychological and physical resources.

3. Respect the patient's way of coping, without making him ashamed or guilty.

4. Be willing to be a target for anger, frustration and aggression, understanding its origin, yet not sanctioning such behaviour.

Case 3

A 51-year-old Greek man with a glioblastoma was referred to the PCS Home Care Program. Communication was impaired by his moderate difficulty with English and due to the deficit associated with his brain tumour. His wife had slight difficulty with spoken English and several other relatives spoke no English at all.

The patient required regular analgesics to control his headaches and was on maintenance insulin for diabetes. Both problems were poorly controlled at home and it appeared that the wife was giving medication very irregularly. Later, it was discovered that the wife feared dependence on drugs, a fear related to her husband's history of morphine abuse following a World War II injury.

The wife was extremely religious and went to mass at the Greek Orthodox Church daily. The Orthodox priest, the only authority she respected, confirmed her belief that it would be better for the patient not to know his prognosis. She frequently took food to Church to have it blessed, feeling that this would do more for her husband than any medication.

On one occasion the patient's sister-in-law arranged to get some holy water from a monastery in Greece and brought it to the hospital to sprinkle over him. When she approached the patient from behind to perform this liturgy, he was startled and struck out at her. She became frightened by his angry behaviour. Those staff members unaware of the significance of the 'holy water' felt somewhat uncertain about the significance of all that had happened.

When the patient was hospitalized, and comatose, the large extended family surrounded his bedside and spilled over into the hall and lounge, significantly infringing on the space and quiet of the other patients and families. The women wept and the men paced the floor. The loss was indeed a community loss.

Comment
Limited English made all communication strained and made it difficult to understand the problems as perceived by this family. Understanding the wife's respect for religious authority, the PCS chaplain contacted the Greek Orthodox priest and explained the difficulty with medication. He was then able to help her understand that God works through doctors, nurses and medications, as well as by miracles. The staff was encouraged to respect her ways of coping, even when her judgement appeared poor.

The staff on the PCU allowed the large family to gather and express themselves in their own way, only interfering when the noise and confusion became troublesome to other patients and families.

Case 4

A 68-year-old Polish-born Jewish woman with a four-year history of colon carcinoma and known pulmonary, abdominal and spinal metastases was referred to the PCS Home Care Program for assistance. Her presenting problem was moderately severe pain in the back, abdomen, chest and especially the right thigh. Multiple adjustments were made in her medication regimen and a course of radiotherapy given. The patient continued to complain of uncontrolled pain though the nurses frequently observed that, while she seemed anxious and fearful, she did not appear to be in physical distress.

Her son-in-law reported that she had always been an anxious, unhappy woman who particularly feared carcinoma of the colon, which had caused the death of another family member. The fear of dying obsessed her. 'I have a slight fever; I know that people die when they have a fever.' When a nurse attempted to interest her in needlework, she replied, 'How can I think of anything, but that I'm going to die?'

Many visits were made by the nursing team, the physician attached to the PCS and a physician friend, yet when the daughter, a psychologist, was reporting a difficult night, she stated, 'I didn't call because no one comes when we call.' When offered a bed in hospital for a period of greatly needed reassurance, assessment and supervision, the patient refused, stating 'You just want to get rid of me.'

She gradually became weaker and died three months later with pneumonia.

Comment

The patient never was pain free during the time she was followed by the PCS, in spite of intensive attempts to control her pain. Her fear of dying influenced all her perceptions. All symptoms confirmed that this fear was justified. The possibility of entering hospital was interpreted as a threat of impending death rather than as an opportunity for assistance.

Zborowski (1952) reported that some Jewish patients he studied tended to be concerned with the symbolic meaning and implications of their pain, whereas other ethnic groups expressed a desire for immediate pain relief. The former group tended to focus on the significance of their pain in relation to their own health and welfare and that of their family. He recommended, therefore, that when caring for Jewish patients one deal with anxieties concerning the source of pain, while in other groups he noted that it was more important to relieve the actual pain.

Schecter (1976) noted that in Jewish families, where each deviation from a child's normal behaviour is looked on as a sign of illness, the child, through conditioning, becomes anxious regarding the meaning and significance of any symptom. He points out that health care professionals with other cultural backgrounds frequently have attitudes toward pain which differ from those held by the Jewish patient. They may feel the patient is exaggerating in describing the pain, either because of undue anxiety or to obtain a secondary gain, such as increased attention from family and staff. The patient, on the other hand, feels that the doctor is ignoring or minimizing his or her suffering. Once again a clearer understanding of the patients' perceptions tends to minimize misinterpretation.

Approaches to bridging cultural and language differences

Several approaches may be of help in these situations.

1. If there is any question concerning clarity of communication, contact a family member who speaks English, or use an interpreter. Learn about the background of the patient, his traditions, his interests, the person he has been.

2. Hold 'family conferences' with significant family members in attendance. These are invaluable in clarifying expectations, allaying fears and improving communications. It is often useful to meet first in the patient's absence, but later the patient should be included so that there can be a sharing of goals and planning.

3. Encourage family and friends to continue to visit, even in the institution. Deal with unrealistic fears and superstitions about the disease.

4. Contact ethnic community service centres which may be able to supply interpreters, assistance with legal issues, social assistance, etc.

5. Identify the staff persons or volunteers whose cultural backgrounds and interests most resemble those of the patient and facilitate their involvement in patient care.

6. Remember that the majority of communication is non-verbal. Even without a common language, a warm smile and a quiet relaxed manner convey a sense of caring and security. An arm around a shoulder or a hand on an arm usually gives support. Watch for non-verbal cues indicating whether such overtures are appreciated or interpreted as an invasion of privacy leaving the patient uncomfortable.

7. Utilize music where appropriate and with skilled support. It provides a unique and powerful tool evoking memories of the past—happy or painful. It crosses all language barriers and is an effective catalyst toward the expression of moods and emotions (Munro and Mount, 1978).

8. Encourage families to bring in favourite foods and specially prepared dishes. Ethnic traditions express themselves in dietary customs. Traditional seasonings can be kept on the ward. Facilities can also be provided to store and reheat food.

9. Look for opportunities to express common values in rituals of worship. A prayer service, for those for whom this would be meaningful, can be held simultaneously in different languages.

10. Where there is no common bond of religious tradition, encourage patients to review their lives and find meaning in their achievements, or in their relationships (Frankl, 1962).

11. Remember that the elderly and the very ill tend to revert to the language and culture of childhood.

12. Organize in-service education programmes which alert staff to significant cultural differences.

13. Make reference materials available to staff, outlining different death rituals and any special care measures for the body at the time of death.

Summary

In many significant cultural areas the patient population of the Palliative Care Service differs significantly from that of the staff. Examples are given indicating some of the difficulties that can arise. Some suggestions are provided indicating approaches toward bridging these differences.

References

Chodoff, Paul (1970). The German Concentration Camp as a Psychological Stress. *Archives of General Psychiatry* **22**, 78.

Frankl, Viktor, E. (1962). *Man's Search for Meaning.* Simon and Schuster, New York.

Hirschfeld, Miriam, J. (1977). Care of the Aging Holocaust Survivor. *American Journal of Nursing* **77**, 1187.

Kalish, R. A. and Reynolds, D. K. (1976). *Death and Ethnicity: A Psychocultural Study.* University of Southern California Press, Los Angeles.

Mufti Abdul Baqui *Muslim Teaching Concerning Death.* A St Joseph's Hospice Occasional Paper.

Munro, S. and Mount, B. (1978). Music Therapy in Palliative Care. *Canadian Medical Association Journal* **119**, 3.

Newman, Lisa (1979). Emotional Disturbance in Children of Holocaust Survivors. Social Case Work. *The Journal of Contemporary Social Work* **60**, 43.

Parrinder, Geoffrey (Ed.) (1971). *Man and His Gods—encyclopedia of the world's religions.* Hamlyn, London.

Schecter, Nathan (1976). Pain and the Jewish Patient. *Journal of Psychology and Judaism* **1**, No. 1, 35.

Zborowski, M. (1952). Cultural Components in Responses to Pain. *Journal of Social Issues* **8(4)**, 16.

The adult patient: reactions to hospice care

John Hinton

The changes in attitude towards the care of the dying seen in the last twenty years include an improved quality of treatment and some renewed ethical questioning. An alteration in values in medical practice is not usually wholly explained by one simple cause. Many factors usually contribute, although a new technique, a pioneer's example, some particular writings or even a particular case may seem to trigger a change in the emphasis in current medical care. One single element has only a transitory effect unless a significant proportion of society is feeling a deeper satisfaction with the current state of affairs. If we consider, for example, the case of the mentally ill, an historical review indicates that advances in treatment with charitable intent or increased freedom granted to the mad often parallel alterations in political or religious climate. Currently, there is considerable concern for people less able to speak up for themselves, the elderly, the mentally handicapped and those with incurable and lethal diseases. In such circumstances it is the special duty of those with the responsibility of, say, caring for the dying, to establish the advances in treatment which give undoubted benefit. Then, if society's interest moves to another fashionable area, there is a hard core of knowledge which will help prevent standards of care falling again to an earlier level of comparative ignorance and neglect.

At present the increased attention paid to the care of the dying has its own momentum. It may well be that a particular pioneer or certain publications initiated a general advance. Hospices, for example, have probably a significant influence on the present climate of affairs. Renewed enthusiasm for looking after incurable and dying people, together with the improvements in treatment available at hospices and some other units have now helped countless patients. But many working in hospices are also aware that more than simple kindness and current enthusiasm are needed to maintain this momentum. We need to learn which policies of care for the dying have proved more successful and can justifiably be recommended to others and which practices should be abandoned. There are times when it seems that you can do almost anything to patients and get away with it as long as you are seen to care. But supposing the attitude of caring wanes and suitable staff replacements are hard to come by—could hospices become the rather isolated, inefficient dormitories for the dying we have seen before? Hence the clear need for critical evaluation of terminal care while the interest is there.

Comparison of types of care

This paper is limited to the presentation of some data I gathered to see if patients dying of neoplastic disease fared very differently when cared for in varying units. Were patients better or worse off if treated by hospice staff as in-patients or out-patients, as compared with those in the radiotherapy wards of a teaching hospital or in a foundation home situated in a large converted house which provided a less formal environment for people with progressive cancer? (Hinton, 1979). At each unit a reasonably matched series of twenty married patients was interviewed. After the patient was seen and assessed, independent information and observations were gathered from the patient's wife or husband. Finally the staff also made their independent assessments.

Before discussing the results it should be noted that the criteria for selection of these subjects included the proviso that they had been in their particular place of care for at least two weeks and that their physical discomfort had been made tolerable. This latter criterion might well be considered to have excluded from consideration a highly important element of hospice technique—the expertise in alleviating pain and other physical distress. Fortunately, these other units were also taking great care to avoid unnecessary suffering and I believe the comparisons made between the units were based on valid samples. This criterion was used because it was, and is, my opinion that continued physical distress plays such a major influence in patients' psychological states that its presence can well swamp the effects of other elements in terminal care. In an earlier study of dying patients, a moderate degree of anxiety readily perceived by the nursing staff was present in only 7 per cent of those without physical distress but manifest in 26 per cent of those whose discomfort was not adequately controlled. Similarly, whereas only 8 per cent of patients free of physical distress showed moderate depression, 35 per cent who still experienced physical distress were moderately or more severely depressed (Hinton, 1963).

The main focus in this paper will be the patients' own opinions, but in case subjective views may be thought potentially misleading, some objective assessments are noted first.

Emotional state

The patient's apparent mood was used as one guide to whether these people appeared to fare better in one unit than another. Rating scales from 1–9 were utilized to assess mood (1 = very elated, 9 = very depressed), anxiety (1 = excessive calm, 9 = agitation) and anger (1 = very benign, 9 = very angry). The ratings were made during my interviews with the patients. Comparable ratings were made by the staff of these units. The information given to me by the patient's wife or husband was also utilized immediately to make ratings. These three sources of assessments showed statistically significant correlations usually about the 0.5 or 0.6 level. The ratings based on the interviews with the patients are illustrated in Fig. 2.5 which compares the four styles of care. In fact, whoever evaluated the patient's mood, the comparisons showed very similar patterns even though scores for each individual did not match perfectly. It is apparent that the hospice in-patients were the most tranquil, the differences often reaching statistically significant levels.

In general, it may be noted that these dying people tended to be a little sad, but marked depression was uncommon. They tended to be anxious, but again they were rarely fearful. Although the anger of dying people is frequently discussed, especially in recent literature with a psychological or psychiatric slant, and undoubtedly some resentful patients do give rise to problems, in these good quality units the patients nearly always spoke and behaved in a way that showed rather less irritation than occurs in normal daily life.

These selected units were of high standard, which is important for at least two reasons. If one wants to discover whether one policy of caring for the dying is better than another, it is misleading to compare units of noticeably different efficiency. The result would be as deceptive as a drug trial in

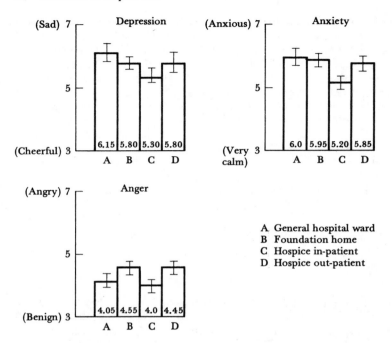

Fig. 2.5   Patients' mood assessment in four types of care. Data given as mean ratings with standard error of the means.

which the optimum dose of one drug was compared with an inadequate dose of another. Another reason for selecting well-run units is to give each policy of care a fair chance of showing what it *can* contribute. Although it emerged that evaluations of these units did differ in some respects to a statistically significant degree, it was also apparent that these different ways of looking after the dying each met with a considerable degree of success. Such results should invite someone to enquire further and determine whether particular ways of care are more suitable for certain types of patient. This is, after all, what general practitioners and others are doing intuitively for much of the time when they refer their patients. Perhaps it would be as well, however, also to warn against using these encouraging results as a basis for complacency. Surveys of the more general care of dying people show that very many do not necessarily get such efficient, sympathetic professional care. They may well continue to experience physical distress and to suffer in mind and body (Cartwright *et al.*, 1973).

Patients' general opinion on their care

Having noted briefly what people thought of the mood of these patients, we shall consider the patients' own views on the treatment they received. Their satisfaction or dissatisfaction with their care will initially be presented in a similar quantitative way to the mood assessments. Using rating scales of 1–9 again (1 = praise, 9 = censure) the four units can be compared for the different aspects of care. The results are shown in Fig. 2.6, based on the comments made by the patients to the interviewers. It can be seen that there was positive approval of nearly all aspects of care. Particular praise was expressed for the staff themselves but the patients were not quite so satisfied with their communications with the staff.

A General hospital ward   C Hospice in-patient
B Foundation home   D Hospice out-patient

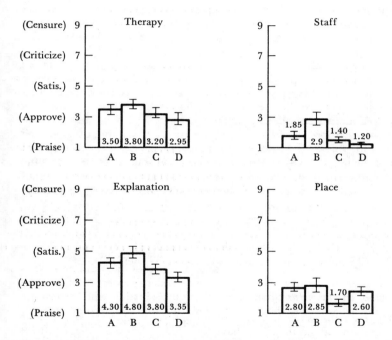

Fig. 2.6 Patients' opinions of four types of care. Data given as mean ratings with standard error of the means. (By permission of *Lancet*.)

In general, comparison between units gave a similar picture to that indicated by the mood assessments; there was a tendency for the groups who were found to be more settled emotionally to give more praise for their care. Patients looked after by the hospice staff tended to express the greatest approval. It is noteworthy, however, that the two criteria of mood and the patients' opinions of their care did not give entirely parallel results when comparing the hospice in-patient and out-patient services. The hospice in-patients tended to be more tranquil than the out-patients. Nevertheless, the hospice out-patients gave slightly greater praise for their treatment, except for the actual location of their place of care which was affected by the level of their own home accommodation. In some circumstances, therefore, treatment at home is highly approved even if there is less emotional calm.

Other people also judged the patients' opinions of their care. Assessments by the staff gave parallel results although the differences between the units often did not reach statistical significance. Similar ratings applied to the patients' approval or criticism of treatment as reported by wife or husband gave over-all results which again matched those based on the patients' direct comments to the interviewer. It transpired, however, that comparing the individual scores given by raters gave correlations in the region of 0.4, lower than the intercorrelations for mood ratings. Following this degree of statistical discrepancy up a little further showed an interesting but understandable clinical side-light. It must be apparent that rating feelings-or opinions according to numbers on a scale of 1–9 is crude enough to produce some variation between observers. In addition, discrepancies may also arise because different observers gain different impressions from patients. When patients' opinions of their care were studied in association with aspects of their personality, as described by their spouses, a cluster of correlations emerged. They indicated that more critical views of treatment were held by patients described as being less satisfied with their lives, more nervous, more indecisive or less able to cope with problems. But these correlations were apparent mainly via the wife's or husband's report of the patient's opinion and rarely came from the patients' comments to interviewer or to staff. In fact, in one item the staff ratings indicated indecisive people showed more approval of their place of care ($r = 0.26$, $p < .05$) while the spouse rated them as more critical ($r = 0.29$, $p < .05$). It seems that when a husband or wife has established a pattern of apparent dissatisfaction, or incompetence, this reaction tends to colour the marital relationship right to the end. The same attitude was not necessarily conveyed to the staff who cared for them.

Patients' views on physical treatment

Quantitative comparisons of the degree of approval expressed by the four groups of patients about their care have their value, but the patients' direct comments have their own impact. Isolated remarks should be interpreted with caution, however, because individuals vary so much, especially when they may be experiencing considerable emotional stress.

The quantitative approach to the physical aspects of medical and nursing treatment the patients received (illustrated in Fig. 2.6) showed no statistically significant difference between units in the opinions the patients expressed to the interviewer. This was not surprising because the units were all of a good standard. It was my general impression that nearly all of the fatally ill patients who had been cared for in these units for a week or two had any physical distress made tolerable; this was certainly the case in the patients studied. According to the views reported through the spouse, one unit did less well, but this isolated finding needs cautious interpretation, especially when we have noted that marital interaction may have some influence on reported opinions.

The qualitative approach to the patients' opinions depends on some of their remarks noted during our assessment interviews. The commonest expression by patients in all units was to say the staff were 'doing their best' or 'doing all they can'. These comments would often show a realistic insight—'I know they're doing their best for me, the medicine here is doing me very well. I've had practically every treatment I can'. Some views expressed the common level of sincere appreciation—'As soon as you feel anything it's coped with'. Occasionally an underlying regret was voiced—'Sometimes I'm disappointed—I don't know their capabilities. I wish the treatment had made me well'. A swing between hope and disappointment about cure occurred a little more commonly in the acute hospital wards—'There's a march of science—I don't give up hope. They try all these things', and another patient said 'I haven't had treatment—just pills and they've given me 3 pints of blood. I hope and believe they're doing their best'. Such views denoted a slightly different emphasis in these wards than in the hospice or home. There can be infinite debate on the benefits of sustaining hope of improvement compared with the advantages of recognizing the need to accept that life is coming to an end. The patients did not indicate a uniform preference for either policy.

Patients' views on their places of care

The fourth histogram in Fig. 2.6 indicates the general approval of these four dissimilar settings. The recently built hospice designed for the specific purpose received a higher degree of praise which, according to the ratings, was statistically significant. The histogram is based on the patients' words direct to the interviewer. Their opinions as conveyed by relatives or nurses were parallel. The patients' views as passed on by wife or husband had a wider range and indicated significantly less approval of the foundation home, although the over-all opinion was favourable. It was easy to see that although the conversion of a large, pleasant house with character can have its attractions as a home for the care of very ill people, a number of design features were inconvenient for nursing.

For all units the individual comments by patients were predominantly those of approval such as the frequent 'This is a marvellous place' or 'It's a nice place'. There was some variation in the flavour of the opinions between the acute hospital wards, the home, the hospice and the hospice domiciliary service. The hospital once again attracted the comments as a place where patients might receive treatment towards cure—'. . . the only way they'll make me better'. As this centre provided a continuity of care for patients since the earlier stages of their illness, the patients would express their sustained faith and loyalty, 'I think (this) is the best hospital, I'd recommend it to any one'. But for some patients being in hospital was just an unfortunate necessity—'I'd rather be here, I can't stand my husband's misery at seeing he could do nothing for me'. One man longed to be away—'I've got to be here while I'm like this. I want to see sky and garden and green trees.'

The foundation home received considerable but sometimes qualified praise, often 'I like it here', 'It's quite nice' or 'It's a wonderful place for the type'. One or two people in certain rooms felt isolated—'At the (other) hospital there was always someone in the room at night'. There were occasional remarks with a direct bearing on the important topic of patients' reactions to entering a place of care where less attention is focused on curative treatment. They indicated a gradual coming to terms with their situation—'Being somewhere like this is something I felt wasn't for me. I still tolerate it . . . it's not ingratitude.' Another lady said 'There was more variety of people at the other hospital but this has worked out better. I first thought I'd been brought here to die and left.' It is apparent that a proportion of patients were prepared to consider consciously the implications of being transferred away from an environment of hoped-for curative treatments. Entering a place where the emphasis was on care rather than cure potentially implied a message. It may well be important to shape and use the way that message about care-giving is conveyed to the patients, especially when they are about to enter the unit. At least those who arrange admission and the staff of the units should consider the fact that many patients will appreciate or perhaps magnify the implications behind their transferral to a different place of care. One explicit statement from a hospice patient indicated that some people can regard it positively. 'It's been wonderful. I made my own doctor promise that when things got too bad I'd be sent to (this hospice) and they'd put me nicely to rest.' Not everyone reaches that state of mind before being admitted, of course.

The hospice, like other units which care for dying patients, could be a very reassuring place; 'I'm very happy here' or 'It's unique—out of this world'. These comments conveyed that the 'place of care' was not necessarily thought of in a limited sense of the architecture or the facilities. Patients, and probably the staff, consider the whole milieu. The patients' direct comments about staff will be considered shortly, but when they spoke of the place where they were receiving care they also thought of the prevailing atmosphere. A place had a morale, reminiscent of certain sea-going vessels which have, say, a reputation as 'a happy ship'. Now and then patients contrasted their present care with previous places of treatment where the impersonal contacts with patients, through understandable staff pressures and problems, could have unfortunate consequences. As a hospice patient recounted 'I have confidence in this hospital. In (the other) hospital, the first night in, the chap in the next bed died in the night. I heard this thud—terrible. These characters said "God, he was heavy". It was the callousness of it all that upset me.'

The domiciliary and out-patient service run from the hospice gave rise to comments about the hospice, usually positive, and the patients' own homes. Given the help and support they had, most patients approved of this type of care—'I wouldn't want to be in hospital unless doctor said it was necessary'—or made clear their wish to stay in familiar surroundings—'I don't want to come in. I don't want to leave home.' It was not universal, however, and occasional comments reflected the need or desire for more continuous professional care—'Sometimes this week I would have preferred hospital. My wife's not getting any rest.' It was a question of judgement of whether the benefits and disadvantages of home care were sufficient to outweigh those of being an in-patient—'I'd rather be at home than at B . . . Hospital, but it's a bit much at home.' The freedom of home and the avoidance of unnecessary separation were appreciated—'I like to listen to music and do tape-recording; I have the dog.' Many will have noted that some patients may say more about separation from their pets than from people. Separation from people, from loved things and from familiar belongings is an ingredient of dying. Being allowed to die at home may relieve premature partings.

Patients' views on staff

As already noted and illustrated in Fig. 2.6, patients expressed high praise for the staff, especially those at the hospice and the general hospital. Superlatives were common, criticism rare—'They've got something to give—happy in the service of Christ.' It was noticeable that patients' comments on treatment were never uniform for any unit. A patient might express an opinion about one unit that might to us seem even more applicable to another; but it is the patients' views being considered, not ours. For instance, that last quotation referred to the staff in the acute hospital ward and not the hospice which had an overt allegiance to Christianity that it did not impose on others. Throughout, there were comments on the nurses' kindness and how much the staff tried to help the patients.

In recent years observers have often described or commented adversely on the care of the dying in a general hospital ward because it might be perfunctory when acutely ill patients are given priority. These patients in the radiotherapy wards did not describe such a picture. This serves as a reminder that an attitude often occurring in a particular setting need not be a necessary part of that setting. If and when deficiencies in care are found in a certain type of unit, it may imply that those aspects of care require improvement, perhaps through education. It does not necessarily mean that such units are quite unsuitable. It is possible that the staff of a successful hospice, for example, may pass on its success by educating the staff of less effective units about particular aspects of treatment. It does not follow that we should plan that all fatally ill people are looked after in hospices. Many patients were well pleased with general hospital care while their lives were coming to an end. Some spontaneously rebutted hackneyed criticisms—'Regimentation's improved since I was last in hospital. People are very nice indeed, helpful and with patience.' 'They can't do enough for you' said another. It is as well to remember that patients are as alert at assessing staff as vice versa, knowing what to look for and, fortunately, in these examples usually came up with favourable judgements—'The staff are marvellous with patients, no undercurrents between people.' Evidently dying people can receive good care in a ward where other patients are at an earlier stage of illness and some are being cured.

The foundation home staff received over-all approval but with slight reservations apparently due to their shortage of time with the patients. 'They're very, very good' was a repeated comment, but also—'They don't seem to have the time. They're awfully good but can't give that little bit extra. I just saw the doctor for a couple of minutes.' Another patient felt the same—'They're dedicated people—I think they're over-taxed here—they're in a hurry, have to rush on.' The practice at this home when it was being assessed was for two doctors to visit regularly while they were also engaged in other medical practice; there was no resident doctor. This plus the fact that the nurses were also kept busy were relevant material reasons for limited time with patients. Evidently these dying patients sometimes thought that more satisfactory care would come if the staff had more than the minimum necessary time to organize and conduct the practical procedures of treatment. Things are not always as simple as they seem, however, and if people hesitate to get involved in awkward discussions with incurable people, the atmosphere of bustle and business may be maintained as protection.

The hospice staff received the highest praise. Various factors contributed to this. The promptness of attention was appreciated—'They've done a lot for me; here they do things straight away.' In addition to the gratitude for efficient care was another element, the feeling of being welcome—'We're all one happy family—a welcome as you come in. I've never seen anything like it.' The reception of the patients on entering the hospice helped them cope with the sense of rejection some patients had when a previous hospital no longer provided in-patient care.

The patients' sense that the staff want to care for them and the feeling of belonging extended to their out-patient care at home 'They've been very nice, most patient. I feel one of the family. Bringing people here (to the clinic) by car, very nice of them.' Patients maintained confidence in the adequacy of home care when they could rely on people they liked—'visited by the nurses, got somebody at the back of you. We like them very much, they're so kind.' Their approval ranged from the ordinary to the supernatural—'very homely' to 'angels'.

Patients' views on communication with staff

Communication between staff and patients about their conditions received, as shown in Fig. 2.6, less approval than other elements of care. Columns C and D in that figure represent the hospice in-patients and out-patients while A and B represent the other units where the staff were less ready for full discussion of the nature of the disease and its likely outcome. The patients who could more easily have frank conversations with the staff about their conditions showed significantly greater approval; this result is discussed more fully in another paper (Hinton, 1979). It may seem that this was a 'halo' effect whereby the more patients liked the staff the more satisfied they were with their mutual discussion. It is appropriate to note straight away that this simple explanation is insufficient. Further analysis of the available data did not show a neat correlation between speaking openly with people and liking them. It is a complex matter involving the willingness to listen to painful feelings, the desire to protect others from hurt and other elements of human interaction. It needs much more study.

The patients' comments about communication could not be fitted into one general principle. The one simple observation which can be made is that in these particular circumstances no patient criticized the staff when they had been frank with them. Open conversations about the patient's condition tended to occur more often at the hospice but they were not confined to this unit. Comments of the patients at the hospital include 'I'm glad I had a conversation with Dr B. It helped that he didn't just say it would be all right. I wanted to know', and 'I've spoken to Dr H. They've told me what I want to know, Dr J. is always optimistic, of course.' Note again that the patients assess the qualities of the staff. Remarks from hospice patients included 'I asked the doctor here and she said it was cancer and really I felt better. I'd got the idea, you see, and I wanted it straight out; it was better than lying awake worrying,' and 'You know what doctors are like, you don't seem to get an answer. Not like that now, I've talked to Dr D., taken it as far as I could.' An out-patient commented 'The biopsy showed malignancy, the doctor told me. I'd far rather they told the truth, it would be humiliating otherwise. They've been frank.' In recent years an increasing proportion of patients have an understanding and knowledge of malignant disease; this trend to greater general knowledge needs to be taken into account in our discussions with patients.

Those who had frank discussion approved. Some of those who had encountered reticence were critical. For instance, 'The first time they said it wasn't anything but wouldn't let me go. Then they told my husband and he told me it was a form of cancer they can treat. Apart from my husband and mother no one will talk about it—seems funny to me', and another commented 'It would be a bit better if they came out into the open a bit more.' The staff were watched for clues—'If they don't tell me I'll think the worst and wouldn't trust the doctors. I watch doctor's expressions.' Even if staff did not consciously communicate, some apparently did so unconsciously. Patients spoke of recognizing prevarication—'Doctor said I had a shadow on my lung—no one's really said—they keep it hush-hush.' Others noted there might be some significance in a degree of avoidance by staff—'There never seems to be any time'. These people could also recognize and perhaps collude in the subtle ways of keeping patients and staff at a distance—'You don't ask your doctor, do you? It's not the done thing.' Only one of these examples occurred with hospice staff, but such opinions were not uncommon in the other units.

The simple model of frankness approved, reticence disapproved, did not apply throughout. In this field of work things are rarely that easy. In all units there were examples where the staff's reticence about the patients' state was approved. A patient at the hospital said 'Doctor just tells me what treatment they plan. I don't want to dwell on my illness; what's to be will be.' A woman in the foundation home was more explicit 'Doctors don't want to talk. Sometimes I don't know whether I want them to really. I wouldn't mind—I'd want them to tell me if it's good but I'm not sure if I want them to say if it's not.' Some hospice in-patients felt the same—'If they've done their job that's all I need to know', so did a patient at home—'I don't want to know too much—I'd be scared inside'.

Even the apparent approval of frankness has its hesitations and likewise when staff are criticized for reticence there are often ambiguities in the situation. A lady who approved of the doctor's explanation nevertheless said 'Before they told me it was inflammation of the bowel and they told my daughter it was cancer. Here they told me it was cancer—it shook me; I had guessed before.' One man also had his reservations although approving in principle, 'I asked the doctor to tell me the whole story, which I rather regretted afterwards, but if they hadn't told me I'd have worried.' The reticence for which staff are often blamed is not necessarily just a confirmation of certain people's autocratic behaviour or their avoidance of discomforting conversation. People who seemed to have mixed feelings about receiving knowledge they might find intolerable occasionally displaced their anxiety and resentment on to the people who held the threatening information. A rather irritable patient whose occasional comments had led others to suspect she might have some idea of the true outlook never asked the staff or confided in them but told me 'You can't speak to these people, they're so important. I don't think I could talk sense to anyone now.' Another lady's account of what happened implied that her own words shaped the uninformative conversations she had with the staff. 'I've asked the doctor if I'm going to get better and they say yes, rather glibly. I want them to say more, but I don't want them to say I won't.' Her question invited so-called reassurance but she was not satisfied with the automatic response when it came.

Having considered the evidence that came to me from these many ill people it is apparent that there is still much to learn about our relationships and communication with dying people. The practice at the hospice clearly met with considerable success. The staff was willing to talk openly to patients when it seemed appropriate. Being prepared to do so, it seemed to follow that neither they nor the patients felt constrained to launch into too much truth at the first possible opportunity. Their judgement over continuing communication appeared to stem from the words the staff and the patients used to each other. Almost certainly there were other cues and intuitive perceptions people use when they are together and aware of each other. When staff were rating the patient's awareness of dying they often commented that the patient seemed to be realizing but had not yet spoken to them about it.

Conclusion

This study has been based on the patients' own views on the effectiveness of some current methods of caring for the dying. Such relatively simple measures can be used to note advances in treatment or monitor the developing proficiency of this craft. Currently, it appears, some hospices have taken the lead in applying the available skills and improving them.

Employing simple ratings of subjective feelings so that they can be handled by current conventional scientific methods may do a disservice to the feelings and to the methods. The present practicable measurements of feelings are often very crude and compare badly with the accuracy attained in some other medical fields. More structural interviews or detailed questionnaires might improve accuracy, but with some dying people such techniques are inappropriate or even unusable. The attempts to measure the thoughts of dying people may distort or limit qualities of subjective feelings which are important when we care for people at a very stressful time of life. Subjective feelings are the province of art as much as science. During my studies at the hospice I have witnessed people practising the art of caring for others, using intuitive perceptions admirably. When the science and the art agree it provides some reassurance that we are on the right path.

This study was possible only through the willing help of people who had a terminal illness, their relatives and the staff of the four units.

References

Cartwright, A., Hockey, L. and Anderson, J. L. (1973). *Life Before Death*. Routledge and Kegan Paul, London.
Hinton, J. M. (1963). The physical and mental distress of the dying. *Quarterly Journal of Medicine* **32**, 1.
Hinton, J. (1979). Comparison of places and policies for terminal care. *Lancet* **i**, 29.

The dying child

Ida M. Martinson

Introduction

The research to be reported here was based on the premise that following the cessation of no longer effective cancer cure-oriented treatment, with death the inevitable outcome, it may be desirable for the child to return to the home environment, and it may be feasible for the family to provide necessary comfort-oriented care with the assistance of a home care nurse and a physician.

In order to determine the feasibility and desirability of a home care alternative for children dying of cancer, it was necessary first to develop and deliver home care services. During the pilot phase, from 1972–1976, we identified the philosophies of comfort care and the policy components necessary for the provision of quality home care, and evaluated the parents' ability to be the primary care-givers for their dying children and the appropriateness of a nurse-directed home care programme. Because there was no existent home care programme that utilized these philosophies and policy components, the research, *Home Care for the Child with Cancer**, was designed with a clinical component that would provide direct home care services and evaluate these services concurrently and after the death of the child. This provision of direct services has been entitled Phase 1.

The research design also called for an institutionalization phase, which was subsequently called Phase 2. During Phase 2, the research staff assisted in the development of home care services in either newly developed or already existent home care programmes in institutions located in the Twin Cities (Minneapolis–St Paul, Minnesota) metropolitan area and throughout the state of Minnesota. Phase 2 also included an evaluation of the development of services provided by those community home care programmes. A third task during the institutionalization phase was to identify all the children served by these community institutions who did not receive home care services and to use these children and their families as a comparison population. In this paper I present some of the findings from Phase I of the Home Care Project.

Groundwork for professional involvement

We first needed to develop ways to educate the health professionals in the community about the possibility of a home care alternative for dying children and about the availability of these services through the Home Care Project. We also wanted to generate referrals from health professionals. Our first activity was to explain the home care alternative and the services available to the paediatric oncologists at the University of Minnesota hospitals. All children would need a physician referral to the research project and the staff would need the physician's assistance in providing the care.

The next group of health professionals we contacted were the nurses at the University of Minnesota Hospitals. Because of the nurses' extensive involvement with the dying children and their families, we believed they could provide invaluable assistance by identifying potential referrals and discussing the home care alternative with the families and physicians. We also hoped that they would become involved in the project as primary home care nurses. Subsequently, an advisory committee was formed which comprised the head nurses, nurse clinical directors and nurse clinical

*Supported in part by Department of Health, Education and Welfare, National Cancer Institute, Grant CA 19490.

specialists at the University of Minnesota Hospitals. They provided educational services to families and suggested referrals. As the project progressed, they also served as consultants to the research staff and gave invaluable feedback on the home care services that were being provided.

The third group of health professionals we contacted were directors of nursing of Twin Cities metropolitan area community health organizations. A community advisory board was formed which comprised these nursing directors, nursing representatives from local and public health nursing agencies, nurse clinical directors from these institutions and a representative from the Minnesota Department of Health. This group informed their nursing staffs and institutions about the home care alternative and served as consultants to the research staff. We hoped that if the results of the research were satisfactory, this group of nurses would later be involved in implementation of home care programmes in their community organizations during Phase 2 of the Project and on a continual basis. Both of these advisory groups met periodically throughout Phase 1 to discuss and evaluate the home care services and the current research.

Patterns of referral

During Phase 1, 64 referrals were made to the research project from physicians practising in nine hospitals and one multidisciplinary out-patient clinic. Thirty-two were referred during the first year and 32 were referred during the second year. At the end of Phase 1, 58 of the referred children had died. Thirty-one (53 per cent) of the 58 children had been treated at the University of Minnesota Hospitals, 12 (21 per cent) had received treatment at the out-patient clinic located in Minneapolis, and 15 (26 per cent) had received treatment at eight other hospitals. Five of these hospitals were located in the Twin Cities metropolitan area, one was in another part of Minnesota, one was in North Dakota and one was in Bethesda, Maryland. Of the 23 physicians who made referrals, 14 (61 per cent) were from the University of Minnesota Hospitals, 1 (9 per cent) was from the St Louis Park Medical Center and 7 (30 per cent) were from other hospitals. The 16 physicians from the University of Minnesota Hospitals and St Louis Park Medical Center were responsible for 74 per cent of the referrals. While several physicians made only one referral, a number of physicians made repeated referrals.

In some instances, a health professional other than the physician was responsible for initiating the referral of the family to the research project. In those cases, the physician was then contacted, the home care alternative was explained and permission to offer services was obtained before the research staff met with the family.

Market penetration

In order to assess the acceptance of the home care alternative by families and health professionals, it was necessary to review the charts of children who died during Phase 1 (July 1976–June 1978) without receiving home care services. We examined the charts of all children who died during the period at the University of Minnesota Hospitals, the largest source of referrals, and made a judgement of the reason the child died in the hospital. During this time, 58 children died while being treated for cancer at the University of Minnesota Hospitals. Of these children, 31 (53 per cent) received services from the home care project and 27 (46.6 per cent) did not receive home care services and died in the University of Minnesota Hospitals. Eleven (19 per cent) of the 58 children were receiving active treatment and would not have been appropriate referrals for home care services. Thus, of the 47 children who might have been appropriate for home care services, 16 were not referred.

Patient and family characteristics

The information obtained from the 58 patient/families who received home care services through the research project provided descriptive characteristics of the families.

Patient age
At death the mean age of the 58 children was 9.3 (SD = 5.5). Children ranged in age from 1 month through 17 years, with a concentration in the age groups 3–5 and 15–17.

Patient sex
Of the 58 children in the study population, 37 (64 per cent) were male and 21 (36 per cent) were female.

Parent age
The mean age of the 57 mothers in the study population was 36.9 (SD = 7.24). Ages ranged from 22 to 58 years. The mean age of the 53 fathers in the study population was 38.6 (SD = 7.51). Fathers' ages ranged from 26 to 61 years. The largest concentration for both mothers and fathers was in the 31–40 age group.

Patient and family residence
Of the 58 families included in the study, 15 resided in the Minneapolis–St Paul metropolitan area, 25 resided in cities and rural areas through Minnesota and 8 resided in neighbouring states of North Dakota and Wisconsin.

Number of family members in household
Three of the 58 families were single-parent families. Two of these were single-mother families and one was a single-father family. In the single-mother families, the mother was the primary caretaker of the family, providing financial, physical and emotional support. In the single-father family, the father lived with his parents; the separated mother returned to assist with the care of the child during the home care period.

Four children in the study had no siblings. The remaining 54 children had a total of 164 siblings, ranging from 17 families with 1 sibling to 5 families with 9 siblings. In addition to families which included the dying child, parents and siblings, there were also instances where grandparents were permanent residents in the home. Households ranged in size from 3 to 12 family members. A large number of families (36) had 0–2 children. Approximately half of the children were 8 years old or younger.

Family ethnic background and race
With the exception of one American Indian parent, all the 111 parents were Caucasian. One parent was Spanish surnamed. This proportion of groups reflects the ethnic mix of Minnesota.

Socio-economic status
We used the Hollingshead Two-Factor Index (Hollingshead, 1957) to categorize the socio-economic status of the 58 families. On the Hollingshead scale, the number I represents the highest social class (in terms of occupation and education) and V represents the lowest. The families included in the study clustered in the lower socio-economic classes, with 81 per cent in classes III, IV and V, and 19 per cent in classes I and II. The dominant social class was IV (47 per cent), followed by III (30 per cent). The 56 heads of households represented all occupational groupings.

Family religion
Fifty-five of the 58 families indicated a religious preference. Among these, both parents in 46 families reported the same religious preference: Protestant (29 families) and Roman Catholic (17 families). In 9 other families the parents reported different religious preferences. On the basis of the mother's stated preference, 6 of these were Protestant families and 3 were Roman Catholic.

Services provided

Role of the family
Parents were considered the primary care-givers of their dying children in the home care model developed by this study. Families provided comfort care rather than cure-oriented care to their children. Each family, including the child if the child were old enough, decided upon its own plan of comfort care in consultation with the nurse and physician. A broad range of possible comfort care measures was available at home to the family, such as the use of intravenous fluids, oxygen administration, gavage feedings and medications such as laxatives, corticosteroids and analgesics. If the family wanted blood-products transfusions, these were available in an emergency room or out-patient clinic. Each family chose the degree of intensity of supportive treatment that it wished to provide at home. Therefore, in some instances the child received intravenous feedings at home and blood-products transfusions at an out-patient clinic to treat the

complications of dehydration and anaemia and also received antibiotics to treat sepsis. In other instances, families, in consultation with the physician, decided not to use these supportive measures. These children were given fluids by mouth as long as possible, the fever was treated with antipyretics and the anaemia was not treated. In almost all instances, the families managed the total provision of this care with minimal physical assistance from the nurses.

Role of the nurse

The nurse served primarily as a consultant to the family, assisting them in assessing the children and in determining and executing a plan of care that would provide for the child's greatest comfort. In addition, the nurse served as a teacher. Parents were initially apprehensive and hesitant to assume responsibility for care that they perceived was the nurses' or doctor's prerogative. The home care nurse reassured the parents that much of the necessary physical comfort care, e.g. mouth washing, providing liquids, and turning and bathing, was care that they had provided for their child at an earlier time. If the parents continued to feel uncomfortable about these basic physical cares, the home care nurse would review them and would also provide instruction regarding new or special techniques that the family had not yet mastered. Parents were thus taught procedures such as tracheopharyngeal suctioning, oxygen administration, administration of intramuscular injections, monitoring of intravenous feedings, administration of gastrostomy tube feedings, irrigation and bandaging of wounds and decubitus ulcers, and administration of urinary drainage equipment. Since the home care nurse was there to assist the family in any manner necessary, nurses also provided direct routine physical care and some specialized cares such as urinary catheterization.

The nurse also procured medical equipment and supplies for the child, making both initial and continuing assessments of the needs for such equipment. She explored the family's community for this equipment and either secured it from readily available supplies or created new supply resources, such as borrowing a suction machine and oxygen mask from a local community hospital or an IV standard from a local nursing home. In addition, the nurse often arranged for delivery of equipment, supplies or medication or delivered them herself. These activities, which we have labelled 'errands', often enabled the family to 'keep going'. Whereas a trip to the chemist at midnight was not pleasant for the nurse, it would have been far more difficult for the parents.

The nurse was in frequent contact with the physician, providing an assessment of the child and family situation and keeping the physician informed. At the beginning of the home care experience, the family, nurse and physician would order the drug with a dosage range, the exact dosage to be decided upon the family and nurse, based upon the child's changing physical condition.

The provision of emotional support to the parents, and in some cases to the dying child, siblings, grandparents, aunts and uncles, consumed a large portion of the time the home care nurses spent during their home visits. Parents often voiced concern regarding the adequacy of the care they were giving their child and needed reassurance that it was equivalent to the comfort care their child could receive in the hospital. They also had many concerns regarding such matters as their family's reaction to the impending death, the many decisions they had to make throughout their child's disease process, the financial problems which resulted, the long-term effects of the child's disease and death on themselves, the siblings and others. The home care nurse served as a counsellor and advocate, assisting the family with financial matters or listening to their opinions when they were dissatisfied with services they had received.

It was also necessary for the home care nurses to describe the dying process to the family, e.g. to explain what possible physical changes or medical complications might occur. This knowledge appeared to help the family prepare for the death. The nurse was available to be present at the death, if the family so wished. Project staff encouraged the home care nurse to attend the child's funeral and to make a follow-up visit within the first month to assess the family's situation. If the nurse believed that the family lacked adequate internal or community support to assist them through the grieving period, she recommended that they seek bereavement counselling or a referral for additional professional assistance.

The services that the home care nurse provided depended upon the individual family's needs and requests. For example, in one instance a 4-year-old boy with rapidly progressing leukaemia returned home to die in the company of his parents, eight siblings and an aunt who was a nurse. The child died one day later. The home care nurse assisted with health assessment, obtained medications, made coroner and funeral arrangements and provided emotional support to the parents and nurse aunt. In another instance, a 15-year-old girl with Ewing's sarcoma returned home to her parents and two siblings. The child had numerous pathological fractures and bed sores. The home care nurse assisted with assessment, physical care and facilitation of the use of equipment and medications. Despite the initial fears of the child and parents, the nurse assisted the family in transferring the child to several different areas of the home, to the girl's great delight. During the three-month involvement the home care nurse offered constant support and encouragement.

Because the child was located at home, because of the nurse's expertise and preparation enabling her to provide comfort care, and because nurses were more readily available and accessible to the family's home, we considered the nurse to be the health care professional responsible for co-ordinating and directing the patient's care. This was always accomplished with the assistance, consultation and support of a physician.

Role of the physician
Physicians were an important component of this model of home care even though they were not as actively involved as the nurses. In all cases the physicians had been involved in the referral to home care. Families

considered the physician's availability for consultation to be important as they called the physician, even if he or she was located at a distant referral centre, to report on their child's health status. The families and nurses, therefore, used the physicians as consultants to answer medical information questions, to make medical assessments based upon the parents' and/or nurses' descriptions of the status of the dying child, and to recommend treatment changes such as medication adjustment and blood-products transfusions. Although almost all contact with the physician was by telephone, children were occasionally examined at an out-patient clinic or doctor's office or by a home visit by the physician.

Utilization of services

We defined the length of home care as beginning after the child's discharge from a health care facility and/or when a home care nurse was available to provide care, and ending at the death of the child. Because a number of the children were re-admitted to the hospital during the home care period and some home care services continued (e.g. home care nurse availability, home care nurses' visits to the child and family in hospital, rented hospital equipment such as beds and suction machines), the child's in-hospital days were also included in the total days of duration of home care. Fifteen (25.9 per cent) of the 58 children had a 'length of stay' in the programme of less than one week, 7 (12.1 per cent) stayed from one to two weeks, and 10 (17.2 per cent) stayed from two to four weeks. Thus, 32 (55.2 per cent) remained in the programme for less than a month. The mean number of days in the programme was 39 and the range was from 1 to 256 days.

The great variability in the duration of home care was due basically to three factors. First were differences among referring physicians; some physicians would refer early when the child was still ambulatory and going to school even though treatment had been stopped. Another physician would wait until that child was confined to bed and home and had begun to exhibit increasing complications of his disease process. A second factor was the normal variability of the disease process in its final stages; and third may be the supportive measures used at home in individual cases.

The very short 'length of stay' of many of the children in the study (less than two weeks) points to the need for home visits within the first twenty-four hours after discharge. Since many families arrange for a discharge immediately after the decision is made to stop treatment, a roster of available nurses is needed so that home care services can start up quickly and begin at discharge.

Number and length of nurse home visits and telephone calls

The mean number of home care visits was 11.7, the median was 7.5, with a range of 1 to 110 visits. The difference between the mean and median was caused by the wide variability in the individual cases served by the study's home care programme. In some instances, the families were very accepting and desirous of frequent nurse contact and assistance. Other families felt capable of independently managing their child's care and stated that they appreciated the nurse's availability and would call upon her if they needed assistance. In a small percentage of instances, the nurse telephoned the family to notify them of her availability and made an appointment for their initial meeting; the next contact was the parents' call to say the child had died or was dying. Thus, in these instances, the nurse's first and sometimes only home visit occurred after the child had died. Another influence on these statistics was the child's disease process. Those children who remained in the study for several months received more visits than those who were in for one month. However, the number of visits usually increased around the time of the child's death.

Because the research staff and the home care nurses were basically committed to returning the control of the child's care to the parents and family, the home care nurses were sensitive to the families' wishes and did not intervene unless they were concerned about the well-being or safety of the child or a family member.

Several of the nurses made daily home visits. While some visits lasted only one-half hour, they often lasted two hours. In some instances, especially at the time of death, visits lasted for hours or even once an entire day.

Nurses and families used the telephone to maintain close contact and often made daily phone calls. In one instance, the nurse visited the family four times in the sixty-seven days of home care service. However, during that time period, she made thirty-eight phone calls, which the mother found very supportive.

The mean number of phone calls was 19.8 which was higher than the number of home visits. The median number of phone calls was 14.5, with a range of 1 to 101. The mean number of hours spent on phone calls was 3.9, the median was 2.4, and the range was 0 to 23.5. Many nurses called daily to check on the condition of the child and family; these phone calls were often brief, 5 to 10 minute calls. Parents remarked that the nurses' 24-hour availability, reinforced by the ready accessibility to her by telephone, was very comforting and provided a sense of security during this stressful time.

Home care nurses were also available to families after the death of the child. They attended the wake visitation, funeral or memorial services and provided bereavement visits. The mean number of post-death visits was 2.3, the median was 2 and the range was 0 to 7.

Family-initiated contacts with nurse during last five days of child's life
There was a total of 103 family-initiated contacts with the nurses during the last five days for the 58 subjects. The mean number of contacts per family during this period was 1.8, with a range of 0 to 6.

Twelve families did not initiate any contacts during the last five days; contacts had all been initiated by the nurse. A few families who returned their child to the hospital before death did not contact the home care nurse, but most families who returned their child to the hospital remained in contact with the home care nurse. If this group of 12 families is excluded from the data, the mean number of family contacts increases only slightly to 2.0.

The primary reason for contacts with the nurse during this period was a change in the child's condition—more than half of the calls (54 per cent) were for this reason. The remainder of the contacts were nearly evenly divided between calls notifying the nurse of death (16 per cent); calls requesting nursing procedures or advice (15 per cent) and 'other' category (16 per cent).

Since change in the child's condition was the most frequent reason given for contacts, we tried to determine what specific changes prompted the calls. A change in the child's neurological status or behaviour was the reason for about 30 per cent of the calls. Respiratory and gastrointestinal tract problems each comprised about 20 per cent of the calls. The remainder of the reasons were fairly evenly divided between fever (19 per cent), bleeding or haemorrhage (9 per cent) and pain (7 per cent).

Only 7 per cent of the changes in condition were in the area of uncontrolled pain. Despite the possibility that some of the calls regarding a child's change in neurological status or behaviour might have been due to uncontrolled pain, the child or family did not verbally identify pain as the reason for the call. This finding suggests good pain control in view of the high priority of need often cited in this area.

Contacts to the nurses regarding nursing procedures needed or advice are broken down as follows: medication, 6 (40 per cent); IVs, 3 (20 per cent); bed or related equipment, 2 (13 per cent); gastrostomy, 1 (7 per cent); urinal, 1 (7 per cent); oxygen, 1 (7 per cent); and Foley catheter, 1 (7 per cent).

Contacts to the nurse for other reasons are broken down thus: related to mechanics of home visits (e.g. dates, time schedules), 5 (31 per cent); progress report or follow-up, 5 (31 per cent); need for support from nurse or home visit, 4 (25 per cent); and ambulance arrangements, 2 (13 per cent).

The above data were utilized in the institutionalized phase and the model of care developed has become part of the health care delivery system in our area. The model has also been followed in Milwaukee, Wisconsin at the Midwest Children's Cancer Center, where 89 per cent of the children have died at home during the past year and a half. Similar programmes have been established in children's hospitals in Los Angeles, California as well as the Children's Hospital in Seattle, Washington. Several hospice groups are beginning to include the care of children in their programmes. The opportunity for parents to care for their child at home appears to be increasingly available throughout the United States.

Acknowledgment

I would like to thank D. Gay Moldow, Research Associate, for major assistance in preparation of this paper and Tim Rand, an undergraduate nursing student, for analysis of data on nurse–family contacts.

Reference

Hollingshead, A. B. (1957). The *Two-Factor Index of Social Position*. Author published.

The family

Thomas S. West OBE and Stephen R. Kirkham

Problems of communication

We have written this paper in two parts—the first an essay on communication and the second a study on insight based on the 591 patients with malignant disease admitted to St Christopher's Hospice, London in 1977.

'The frequent recognition by people that they may well be dying means that the question is not so much "Does the doctor tell?" but "How much do they discuss?" Some said they wanted the whole truth or some explanation. Others wished to abdicate all knowledge and responsibility, or wanted re-assurance, perhaps stating that if the prospects were bad they did not want it said' (Hinton, 1974).

Essay on communication

Introduction

'Doctors, for the most part, are uninterested in disability and dislike the contemplation of mortality . . . whereas their patients have always been more concerned . . . with living, and with its length and with its quality' (MacLean, 1979).

The vexed question of 'telling' cancer patients is frequently discussed. In practice it would seem that more patients are not told or are misled than are properly informed. Identifying the obstacles to good exchange of information and recognizing means of overcoming them could result in an improvement in what is now a sadly haphazard situation.

The question posed is 'Who should tell what to whom—when, where and how?'

Who should tell?

It is commonly expected by both the medical profession and the public that information about the diagnosis and prognosis of cancer patients should come from a doctor. Unfortunately, before a definite diagnosis and an estimate of the prognosis can be made the patient will almost certainly have passed through the hands of many doctors but will have become the responsibility of none.

In the first stages of his disease the patient will have been referred by his own doctor to a large centre for investigations, diagnosis and possible treatment. He begins at an out-patient clinic, and from this starting point he is 'processed' through the haematology, the x-ray, the surgical and occasionally the psychiatric departments which, in turn, take his blood, his films, a biopsy and his security. Not one of these departments will have taken overall control of his care.

In the early stages the doctors may well feel sufficiently optimistic about the outcome to conceal the diagnosis from the patient. In the later stages they feel so impotent that their own denial mechanisms may prevent their re-opening a book which they have (often with the connivance of the family) firmly closed. The phrase 'The doctor said there was nothing more that could be done' may not be a verbatim account of the words used but is frequently an accurate picture of the message transmitted.

If the consultant, holding the results of laboratory tests and x-rays in his hands, is for any reason unable to share them with the person to whom they refer, then he must convey this fact as well as the results themselves to the family physician (Calman and Murdoch, 1974). And if the family physician does not receive clear information on all points, including insight, he should contact the consultant before he makes an appointment to meet the patient.

Occasionally the patient may question other people. These include ward staff, members of his family or even other patients. If doctors have continually failed to take the responsibility of giving to the patient the information that he *wants* and *needs*, they should then be prepared to support the action of those who do have that courage (West, 1978).

'Sick people only become patients when they come under a doctor's care . . . Sometimes, it is the influence of other people and the inherent dignity of their concern that makes the difference between a meaningless and a purposeful death' (Weisman, 1972).

What should be told?

To most people the word 'cancer' conjures up a picture of prolonged, inevitable, painful death—probably taking place in increasing isolation. By using the word 'cancer' or by encouraging the patient to bring it out into the open, most of the fears and anxieties associated with this word can be dispelled.

If, at the time of diagnosis, the word 'cancer' is not used—or at least clearly understood—it will probably be difficult for any doctor to use it until the terminal stage has begun. Unfortunately, it is likely that in the intervening period in ward or out-patient clinic or radiotherapy department the patient will have come to his own conclusions. The barrier being built between doctor and patient is now completed.

The whole truth is seldom accurately told, largely because it is seldom completely known. But to lie is wrong and usually unnecessary. The patient needs to be told three things in words he can understand. He should be told what is wrong with him, what it may possibly mean in the future and what medical science has to offer him (Elland quoted in Duncan *et al.*, 1977). The difficulties of language should be remembered and constant checking, both verbal and non-verbal, should monitor the success of the communication. Some doctors may be thought to tell their patients too much too soon while others may be thought to tell their patients too little too late. Proper communication, at all stages, lies somewhere between these two extremes (McIntosh, 1977).

'Truth, like medicine, can be intelligently used, respecting its potential to help and to hurt. The principal worth in sharing truth is to encourage viable responsiveness between people as long as possible. After we come to terms with talking about death, details such as what to tell, when to tell, how much to tell, and how often and in what form it may be repeated can be arranged for the needs of the individual patient and the compunctions of the survivors. It is as dogmatic and inexcusable to insist upon full disclosure about a deadly disease early in the course as it would be to proscribe any discussion whatsoever' (Weisman, 1972).

To whom should it be told?

It is customary for the diagnosing clinician to inform the family of the results of investigations but, unless the news is good, for the patient to be 'protected' by silence or meaningless words of comfort. 'Only in the area of pediatrics and terminal illness is it customary to ask responsible family members to decide for the patient. Were we to act in accordance with what we profess about psychological processes, we would *first* tell an adult about the diagnosis and plan for treatment. Only then would the doctor, after consultation with his patient, decide what and when to tell the family' (Weisman, 1972). It is hard to believe that it is ever right to tell the family so much and the patient so little that the gap between their insights becomes unbridgeable.

When there is hope of a cure, that hope should be shared. When the disease appears to have escaped control the patient should not be automatically excluded from this new knowledge.

Sometimes, when the bad news has been broken to the spouse the doctor can suggest, before protective denial has intervened, that it might be useful if he came to the bedside and talked with the patient and spouse together. It is doubtful if the doctor should ever agree that the patient should *never* be told, or accept that the patient would 'give up' if he knew.

When should it be told?

The time of diagnosis, not the time of suspicion, would seem to be the appropriate occasion for discussion to take place. Most patients and their families have some idea of the reasoning behind routine investigations—indeed their speculations may be considerably more horrific than the truth. There is an inevitable time of anxiety between test and result and the appointment at the end of this period is crucial. It is now that the doctor holding the cards must decide how the hand should be played.

At this stage, timing becomes extremely important. It may be inappropriate for the hospital doctor to give the patient bad news immediately prior to his discharge unless he is able to follow-up such a critical conversation. If the patient is to be discharged to home or hospice without further insight, then it is the duty of the hospital doctor to pass the burden of communication back to the family doctor along with the responsibility for further care. This also involves the decision as to whether further out-patient appointments are appropriate or merely a farce.

If the patient chooses to deny or suppress the facts, then the next occasion when communication may open up will be when the disease reasserts itself and palliative treatment or symptom control is started. If this opportunity is missed (by either patient or doctor) and symptom control is successful or a remission occurs, it is once more inappropriate to thrust bad news at someone who now feels better rather than worse.

Again, the team must wait. The right time for offering information may not recur until the patient makes a positive move towards knowledge. 'Why am I not getting better?' (or a variation) is the question that indicates the re-opening of enquiry. Questions may now be asked of family, of friends, or ward staff but often not of the doctor. Only if team communication is open will the doctor be aware of the progress in the patient's thinking and be able to respond carefully but openly himself (West, 1978).

How should it be told?
'How the physician responds to the commitment he makes to the dying patient is determined more by his own personality than by the grimness of the diagnosis or the debilitation of the patient. The patient's capacity to face his own imminent death is often underestimated, while the doctor's capacity to face the patient's death is usually overestimated' (Weisman and Hackett, 1962). If the doctor accepts this distinction, he may well find that the patient is unexpectedly well prepared to receive further information. This is the time for the doctor to approach his objective with sensitivity and with strength. Referring to statements made by the patient, his family, or reported by the staff, can be a useful introduction for the doctor. From then on he should plan his communication in stages—answering no more and no less than the questions the patient has asked and be prepared to stop at any one of them if he becomes aware that the patient has, for the time being, received all the information he can contain (Abrams, 1974).

Too often doctors do not watch the effect of their attempts to communicate. In this they resemble efforts to communicate with the deaf or with foreigners when a smile or a repeated 'Yes' is assumed to validate the successful passage of information from the transmitter to the receiver.

Where should it be told?
Information concerning life and death should not be conveyed from a position of superiority. The hospital doctor should not stand at the end of the bed, nor be surrounded by a retinue. Facing the patient and speaking with authority but listening with compassion, the doctor shows his own humanity without losing the patient's confidence in him. Sometimes it is appropriate to have a sympathetic ward sister or senior nurse present—also

sitting. Her presence will often catalyse communication and give both doctor and patient the courage to speak and to ask questions. She will be able to convey to the ward staff and the family what stage communication has reached. Sometimes another member of staff whom the patient knows and trusts, or a member of the family or a close friend can facilitate this encounter of fears with facts. This dialogue may be best undertaken away from other patients and in privacy. But if the doctor is truly concentrating on his target, it is surprising how disturbances (though not the bleep!) will be easily ignored.

It would often seem appropriate for the specialist in the hospital to inform the patient of the diagnosis of his disease and its probable outcome. This must be backed up by a family doctor who has been competently, clearly and quickly informed by the hospital staff of the facts and of the degree of insight they believe the patient possesses. Whether the doctor chooses to tell a member of the family or the patient first is for him to decide. That he should then encourage this information to be shared with the others intimately concerned would seem essential (Feifel, 1977). In the history of this family, surely at no other time can shared knowledge and a united front be more important.

The study on insight

Introduction

Most of the material published about talking to cancer patients is anecdotal, some is opinionated, and even where numerical results are presented the population studied is often self-selected. In particular, there are few figures available on how much insight such patients have and how they obtain their knowledge. This study was undertaken to try to answer these two questions.

Methods

We have analysed the figures for insight for the year 1977. Every patient admitted to St Christopher's Hospice has had an application form filled in by the referring doctor, who may work in a hospital or be a general practitioner. At admission to the hospice, the admitting doctor assesses the degree of insight that the patient shows and records this under 'Insight' in the notes. Occasionally, where a patient has been under the domiciliary team before admission, such an assessment will be made by a home care nurse.

Two sources of information have thus been used. First, we have assessed the amount of information that has been given to the patient about his illness by categorizing the answers given to the question on the application form: 'What has the patient been told about his/her illness?' Secondly, we have taken the degree of insight noted at first contact with St Christopher's.

I. We have divided the amount of information given to the patient by the referring doctor (according to the application form), into eight categories.

1. *Told the diagnosis and the prognosis.* This category includes answers such as, 'everything', 'all about it' and 'fully aware'. For patients who have been told the diagnosis, we have considered that the phrase 'we cannot cure him' gives sufficient idea of the prognosis to merit inclusion here.

2. *Told the diagnosis.* We have included the answers 'yes', 'fully aware of the diagnosis', 'progressing tumour (or growth)' and 'brain tumour'. We have also included a knowledge of cancer in the past, even though there is no stated knowledge of active cancer at the time of referral.

3. *Told partial truth.* This includes such terms as 'tumour', 'growth', 'the original trouble', 'blockage', 'serious incurable illness' and 'poor prognosis'.

4. *Not told, but apparently aware of the diagnosis and/or prognosis.*

5. *Given incorrect or misleading information.* We have included the terms 'wart', 'ulcer' and 'cyst', unless it is definitely stated 'which has spread'. We have also included 'inflammation' and 'chronic infection' here.

6. *Patient evaded discussion.*

7. *Told nothing.* This includes 'no', 'thinks he has (any of 5)' and also 'I think he has guessed' and 'I think he probably knows' as being too uncertain to belong to 4.

8. *Space left blank.*

II. We have also divided the degree of insight noted on first contact with St Christopher's Hospice into eight categories, corresponding as closely as possible with the above and labelled A to H. We have considered the spouse, but not other close relatives, a reliable source of information. The eight categories are as follows.

A. *Knows the prognosis.* This is usually with, but occcasionally without, the diagnosis.

B. *Knows the diagnosis.* A determination to fight or get better does not disqualify from this category.

C. *Has partial knowledge.* This corresponds with 'told partial truth' above.

D. *Suspicious* (for example, depressed or weepy when talking about the illness) or *enquiring* (especially asking direct questions about the diagnosis or prognosis on admission).

E. *Admitted to St Christopher's Hospice for convalescence or treatment.*

F. *Denial of the illness.*

G. *No insight.* This includes 'I have an ulcer' and the relatives saying 'I think he might suspect'.

H. *Insight not revealed.* We have included those patients confused or comatose on admission.

We have allotted each patient to one of the resulting 64 (i.e. 8 × 8) groups. The totals discussed below have been analysed using the χ^2 distribution, using Yates' correction where appropriate.

The results were also drawn up in a grid, to test how *information given* affects *insight possessed* by patients. Categories 8 and H have been excluded.

As noted above, the categories 1 to 7 and A to G have been chosen so that as far as possible successive categories correlate. Thus, we would expect patients to fall along the diagonal A1 to G7.

Results

During the calendar year 1977, 591 patients with malignant disease were admitted to St Christopher's Hospice. Of these, 282 were referred by hospitals and 309 were referred by general practitioners. The assessment of insight was made by a home care nurse in 3 patients. The mean age of those patients referred from hospital was 65.0 years (SD 12.0) and for those referred from general practitioners was 66.5 years (SD 10.9). The two groups were well-matched for sex (Table 2.4) and were also well-matched

Table 2.4 Source and sex distribution of 591 patients with malignant disease admitted to St Christopher's Hospice in 1977.

1977 patients	Hospital	GP	Total
Male	122	132	254
Female	160	177	337
Total	282	309	591

Table 2.5 Duration of illness at time of admission (X^2 = 4.94, DF = 5, not significant).

	0–3 m	>3–6 m	>6 m–1 y^r	>1–2 y^r	>2–5 y^r	>5 y^r
Hospital (282)	37	53	64	53	44	31
GP (309)	28	51	85	56	58	31

for duration of illness at the time of admission (Table 2.5). Analysis of the total numbers of patients falling into each of the 16 groups above (1 to 8 and A to H) showed no significant difference between male and female populations. Only 2 of the 16 showed a difference significant at the 5 per cent level when hospital referrals were compared with general practitioner referrals (Table 2.6). The differences were that there were more patients in category 3 (i.e. told partial truth) referred from hospitals than from general practitioners, and similarly more in category G (possessing no insight) referred from hospitals than from general practitioners. The overall difference is probably not in fact significant.

Table 2.6

Category	Hospital	GP	Category	Hospital	GP
1	39	32	A	51	63
2	68	84	B	57	74
3	59*	44*	C	20	23
4	7	15	D	31	29
5	33	34	E	4	6
6	5	1	F	9	6
7	66	95	G	67*	50*
8	5	4	H	43	58

* Significance $0.01 < p < 0.05$.

Inspection of the grids correlating *information given* with *insight revealed* (Figs. 2.7 and 2.8) shows that the patients falling on the diagonal A1 to G7 possess insight appropriate to the amount of information given. Those lying above the line have less insight than expected, and those lying below the line have more insight than expected. Categories 8 and H, totalling 109 patients, have been excluded as being impossible to assess. In the remaining population of 482, we have found that for neither hospital

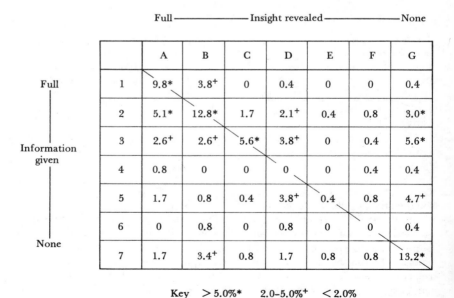

Full ——————— Insight revealed ——————— None

		A	B	C	D	E	F	G
Full	1	9.8*	3.8+	0	0.4	0	0	0.4
	2	5.1*	12.8*	1.7	2.1+	0.4	0.8	3.0*
Information given	3	2.6+	2.6+	5.6*	3.8+	0	0.4	5.6*
	4	0.8	0	0	0	0	0.4	0.4
	5	1.7	0.8	0.4	3.8+	0.4	0.8	4.7+
	6	0	0.8	0	0.8	0	0	0.4
None	7	1.7	3.4+	0.8	1.7	0.8	0.8	13.2*

Key > 5.0%*   2.0–5.0%+   < 2.0%

Fig. 2.7 Patients referred from hospital for whom both information given and insight into illness are known. Percentages, total n = 235.

Full ——————— Insight revealed ——————— None

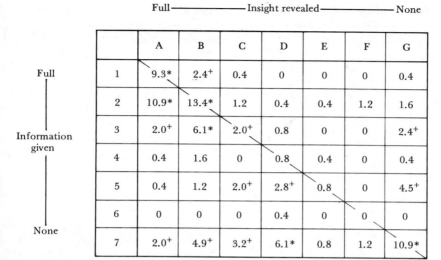

Key > 5.0%*   2.0–5.0%+   < 2.0%

Fig. 2.8 Patients referred from GP for whom both information given and insight revealed are known. Percentages, total n = 247.

referrals (235) nor general practitioner referrals (247) is there a particularly good correlation between what the doctor believes the patient has been told and what the patient actually remembers. Hospitals did slightly better (98, or 41.7 per cent 'correct', i.e. lying on the diagonal line) than general practitioners (92, or 37.2 per cent 'correct'), although the difference is not significant.

The results also show that for patients referred by hospitals, there is an even distribution above and below the line. However, for those patients referred by a general practitioner, a greater proportion lie below the line

Table 2.7 Degree of insight revealed compared with amount of information given. (X^2 = 18.67, DF = 2, p<0.001).

Source of referral	More insight	Equivalent insight	Less insight
Hospital	68	98	69
GP	114	92	41

than above the line (p < 0.001): that is, a highly significant proportion of patients referred by general practitioners show more insight than we were led to expect (Table 2.7). This result was apparently matched by a highly significant difference in the marital status of the two groups (Table 2.8),

Table 2.8 Marital status according to source of referral of 591 patients with malignant disease admitted in 1977 (X^2 = 21.67, DF = 3, p<0.001).

Source of referral	S	M	W	D	Total
Hospital	53	126	86	17	282
GP	30	193	76	10	309

with the 'hospital' group being predominantly single, widowed or divorced, and the 'general practitioner' group being predominantly composed of married people. However, when the marital status of each person in the grids was determined, we found there was a random distribution below and above the diagonal line of patients with spouse and without spouse (Tables 2.9 and 2.10). Thus, the presence of a spouse at home does not appear to help a patient towards greater insight.

A pilot study carried out on 36 patients with malignant disease who were

Table 2.9 Significance of spouse as source of information. Patients referred by hospitals.

	More insight (%)	Equivalent insight (%)	Less insight (%)
M	42.6	50	39.1
S/W/D	57.4	50	60.9

Table 2.10 Significance of spouse as source of information. Patients referred by general practitioners.

	More insight (%)	Equivalent insight (%)	Less insight (%)
M	67.5	59.8	63.4
S/W/D	32.5	40.2	36.6

in-patients at St Christopher's Hospice on one particular day, has shown that 23 had good insight as to their diagnosis. Of these, 13 said they had been told by their hospital, 2 by a member of their family and 2 by a member of the staff at St Christopher's. We could not assess the source of information in the other 6 patients. None of them had been told the diagnosis by their general practitioner.

Discussion

Reporting and recording significant conversations that staff have with patients about their illness should be included as an important part of their management. This is rightly so, as a mistaken belief that a patient knows more—or less—than he does can lead to serious blunders and distress. In this survey, we have studied only one aspect of communication in cancer patients—the degree of agreement between doctor and patient as to what the patient has been told. Most authorities agree that non-verbal communication is an important means by which information is conveyed to the terminally ill. However, we have had to disregard it. We have also had to assume that the referring doctor has an infallible memory for conversations that have taken place some time earlier. We can see no reason why these assumptions should not affect our two groups equally, and so not affect the significance of our results.

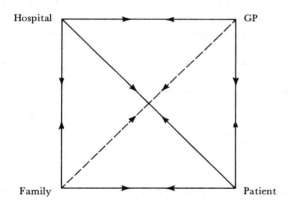

Fig. 2.9 'Square of commmunication'.

There are various routes by which medical information may reach the ultimate target—that is, the patient. The ultimate source of most of this information is a hospital (Fig. 2.9). In the case of general practitioner referrals, a highly significant proportion of patients appears to be gaining insight without that doctor's knowledge. This difference between hospital referrals and general practitioner referrals cannot be explained on grounds of age, sex or duration of illness. Nor, interestingly, does it seem that the spouse (or, presumably, the rest of the family) is a significant route by which patients learn the diagnosis. It appears that patients at home do *not* talk about their diagnosis.

Our results therefore indicate the following.

1. A member of hospital staff is the source of most of the information that our patients have about their illness. Our findings here disagree with those of Cartwright *et al.* (1973) who carried out a retrospective study on the relatives of people who had died of a wide variety of conditions. They found that approximately equal numbers of patients with neoplasms had been told the prognosis by hospital staff and by general practitioners. However, the number of patients who knew, but had been told by 'no one' was greater than in either of these two groups. All three of these groups together were easily outnumbered by those who knew nothing.

2. Hospital doctors do not include in their discharge summaries a statement of what the patient has been told about the illness. This agrees with the findings of Calman and Murdoch (1974), where only 3 out of 50 discharge summaries contained this information. We believe that this should be a very important part of the summary.

3. General practitioners appear to fail to a very significant extent to discover how much patients know about their malignancies, and probably therefore are unable to cope properly with any mental distress arising from that knowledge, or lack of it. This is surprising, as it is widely stated that general practitioners know their patients better than do their colleagues in hospitals and therefore communicate better.

There is obviously a great need for further research to be carried out into the whole subject of talking with dying patients. In particular, we should know whether people believe they are better off for being told the position, whether they cope well with such knowledge and whether, given the choice, they would have had things any different.

MacLean (1979), reviewing the literature, indicated that between 70 per cent and 90 per cent of patients either would like to know of a diagnosis of a malignancy or thought that people in general should be told of such a diagnosis.

To contrast with this, Oken (1961), reviewing the literature dating back a decade and also publishing his own results, suggested that some 70 to 90 per cent of American physicians had a policy of either usually or always keeping the diagnosis from the patient. Papers published more recently, however, show a marked change in attitude. Rea *et al.* (1975) found that 61 per cent of 151 physicians believed that patients *must* be told of terminal illness, and Carey and Posavac (1978) found that 71 per cent of 45 physicians would take the initiative in revealing the terminal condition. Of our patients, we would consider that 44 per cent to 64 per cent have been given 'good' information (categories 1 + 2 ± 3) and 48 per cent to 57 per cent have 'good' insight (categories A + B ± C). These figures agree approximately with those of Cartwright *et al.* (1973) who, in the study described above, found that 30 per cent to 50 per cent of patients who died with neoplasms were thought by relatives to have known what was wrong.

Davies (1973) points out that for any procedure requiring a patient's consent (presumably including all operations), 'there can be no true consent without knowledge, (and) there must in those cases be no withholding the truth, whether the patient has specifically asked for it or not'. Of our 591 patients, 461 (78 per cent) had had some form of operation (diagnostic, curative or palliative) for their malignancy. This theoretical legal requirement does not therefore appear to be followed in widespread clinical practice.

Henderson (1935) exhorted his readers to 'try to do as little harm as possible . . . in treatment with words, with the expression of your sentiments and emotions'. Whether or not we have read these words, we all as doctors have an innate reluctance to do anything which *we think* might harm the patient. The fear of immediate harm, even though mild, will bring out this reluctance more than a distant, less certain but potentially more serious harm. We resemble Isaac Asimov's telepathic robot 'Herbie' who had built into his positronic brain the overriding command of the First Law of Robotics: 'A robot may not injure a human being or, through inaction, allow a human being to come to harm'. This command, too, set up a strong potential against causing mild immediate distress at the expense of later, serious distress (Asimov, 1968).

If we do not tell our patients the truth, perhaps without necessarily being asked, our patients may later ask *why* they have not been told. Such a question is virtually impossible to answer to the patient's satisfaction. One patient (D.M., male, 56) has asked us, in a tone of disbelief, 'Do you mean to say my family and the nurses all knew I had cancer, and I didn't? They must have been laughing their bloody heads off.' The implied question, 'Do you think that's fair?' can only be answered 'No'.

If we decide 'not to tell' we should ask ourselves 'why not?' If we cannot answer that to our own satisfaction, perhaps we should think again.

References

Abrams, R. D. (1974). *Not Alone with Cancer*, p. 44. Thomas, Springfield, Illinois.

Asimov, I. (1968). Liar. In *I, Robot*, p. 92. Panther, London.

Calman, K. C. and Murdoch, J. C. (1974). What does the general practitioner want to know about the cancer patient? *Lancet* ii, 770.

Carey, R. G. and Posavac, E. J. (1978). Attitudes of physicians on disclosing information to and maintaining life for terminal patients. *Omega* 9, 67.

Cartwright, A., Hockey, L. and Anderson, J. L. (1973). Awareness and information about death and illness. In *Life before Death*, p.163. Routledge and Kegan Paul, London.

Davies, Lord Justice E. (1973). The patient's right to know the truth. *Proceedings of the Royal Society of Medicine* 66, 533.

Duncan, A. S. Dunstan, G. R. and Welbourn, R. B. (1977). *Dictionary of Medical Ethics*, p.330. Derton, Longman and Todd, London.

Feifel, H. (1977). Discussing diagnosis with patients. In *New Meanings of Death*, p.99. McGraw-Hill, New York.

Henderson, J. J. (1935). The physician and patient as a social system. *New England Journal of Medicine* 212, 819.

Hinton, J. (1974). Talking with people about to die. *British Medical Journal* 3, 25.

MacLean, U. (1979). Learning about death. *Journal of Medical Ethics* 5, 68.

McIntosh, J. (1977). *Communication and Awareness in a Cancer Ward*. Croom Helm, London.

Oken, D. (1961). What to tell cancer patients. *Journal of the American Medical Association* 175, 1120.

Rea, M. P., Greenspoon, S. and Spilka, B. (1975). Physicians and the terminal patient. *Omega* 6, 291.

Weisman, A. D. (1972). *On Dying and Denying, a psychiatric study of terminality*. Behavioural Publications, New York.

Weisman, A. D. and Hackett, T. P. (1962). *The Dying Patient*. Forest Hospital Publications 1.

West, T. S. (1978). In-patient management of advanced malignant disease. In *The Management of Terminal Disease*, p.139, Ed. by C. M. Saunders. Edward Arnold, London.

3
A philosophy for dying

The Rev Canon John Austin Baker

I want to reflect on certain questions which some might regard as either taboo or irrelevant in the context of hospice work. These are the questions about what, if anything, happens after physical death. Does the story go on after the chapter we help to write is finished? Does it make any practical difference to our work here and now, whether it does or not?

There are good reasons for ruling these subjects out of order. Everyone who comes into a hospice must be equally welcome, equally respected in terms of what they are as unique individuals who have written their own story. Any suggestion that they should be put under pressure, however kind, to modify their beliefs in any direction is quite unacceptable, above all at such a time. Moreover, in a society that is both fundamentally secularized and religiously pluralist, any other attitude would make it impossible for the hospice to serve the commodity as a whole. Dying is a universal human necessity, and our job is to help the dying person make it not just something to be endured but, as far as can be, a creative, positive, dignified and worthy part of their total living. We are in a human, here-and-now relation with them; and we have to contribute our present skills, respect, loyalty and love to help make the best of something we share with them—our mortality.

The same need for everyone, so to speak, to start level applies within the staff of a hospice as well. It would be intolerable that those who do not believe in anything beyond should not be able to give what they have as part of the team—and what they have may be more than others, for they may take dying with greater seriousness. One ought certainly not to risk anything which might tend to divide one worker from another. Whatever the private convictions of any individual, there must be an agreed basis for their professional collaboration; and any attempt, therefore, to inject inevitably disputable areas of belief into the content of professional activity and attitudes is likely to be divisive and harmful.

Finally, as the hospice movement spreads all over the world, and is taken up in widely differing societies and cultures, the members of which may adhere to very different religious faiths and conceptions of human nature and destiny, it must become more problematic and possibly unhelpful to raise such matters.

All this is very much the accepted thinking at the moment. Yet it seems to me to overlook one or two very significant facts. Despite the steady increase in the number of people in the world who hold a humanist and strictly this-worldly view of life, whether based on Marxism or on some other philosophy, the large majority do still think in terms of some sort of continuance after death. The particular form of continuance will vary considerably with different religious or world views. For many it will be a belief held without belonging seriously to any religion or recognizable school of thought—simply a deep but vague and unexamined assumption within their own culture. Nevertheless, as anyone who has done much pastoral or counselling work will know, the belief (or perhaps it would often be better described as a feeling or intuition) that our visible, physical life is not the whole of our personal history is exceptionally tenacious. It survives not merely the powerful intellectual arguments constantly launched against it (which in both their popular and more sophisticated forms are again and again dismissed with what must seem to the arguers exasperating obstinacy) but also, more significantly, the actual agonizing doubts within the believer's ówn mind. It is hardly exaggerating to say that many people, in Western society especially, simply refuse to accept the verdict of their own rational mind on the probabilities in this matter.

This situation suggests two thoughts for those engaged in the care of the dying. First, the majority of those to be cared for will have some sort of conviction that bodily death is not the end of personal existence. Secondly, this conviction has very deep roots in human physical make-up. I find it hard to explain belief in survival except in terms of some almost structural feature of human nature. For one thing, as we saw, it seems unaffected when the rational grounds for it are cut away. The guess has been hazarded that primitive peoples came to believe in survival because they still saw in dreams those who had died, and did not realize that dreams are not the same in character as waking seeing. But if this is true, it is also true that when the real nature of dreams was understood, it made no apparent difference. It is even more certain that belief in future existence has been supported by religious authority, particularly that of sacred texts (the Bible, the Koran, etc.). But where the credibility of the Christian Bible, for example, has been rejected, there has by no means been an equal rejection of belief in life after death. In a negative sense it is worth noting, too, that when, as in Ancient Israel for most of its history, it was religious orthodoxy that repudiated a future life, the effect was very often either to drive belief in such a life underground or to drive believers away to other, less austere religions.

What is this deeply ingrained conviction? Philosophically (using that word in a wide, popular sense) it seems to me to be at all periods bound up with that crucially significant human attitude, *the reflective awareness of Time.* It is, I believe, true to say that human personality cannot develop in any coherent way until this awareness exists. If we ask why our conscious memories go back only so far, normally not beyond about 3 years of age, sometimes no further than 4, the most probable answer is that until we can look backwards and forwards, and relate past to present and future, we have no framework in which to make sense of our memories, and so they remain lost in that storage we call the 'unconscious'. We need to be able to say to ourselves 'This has happened before'—the seaside, a festival, a birthday—over a reasonably long perspective before we begin to become aware of our life as a story, and so to be conscious of the fact that to some extent its development is in our own hands. What happens to this sense of Time, what feelings and values get tied up with it, are decisive for the kind of person we become.

Not for nothing are the poets obsessed with this theme of Time and all its complex variations. Time is the very stuff of personality. Whether we are the passive victims of Time, swept along by it like a stick in a stream; or for a while, anyway, the victors over it, using it to the full to do what we want; or simply stranded souls who have lost touch with Time and wasted it in a life of non-experience; or, as with most people, can look back on a life that is a mixture of all these things; the tone of our character as we come to die will be determined principally by the balance struck within our souls between them. 'I wish . . .'; 'If only . . .'; 'I might have . . .'; 'I've had a good life . . .'; 'Nothing ever . . . no one ever . . . now it's too late'; 'I would have liked . . . but I mustn't grumble'; 'It's nice to think . . .'; 'There are things . . .'. All these familiar phrases are attempts to come to terms with a closing story, to be able to feel that in the end we can make some sense of it all, be not wholly displeased.

It is important to be able to do this for two reasons, closely linked with each other. The first is concerned with value; we do not want to feel that our life has contributed nothing, been worthless. We have after all put into it everything; that is what we were—whether we could have been more is irrelevant, that is all that in the end we had to give. The second is concerned with integration: we want to bring into some sort of resolution and harmony the patchy, fragmented, morally, emotionally and aesthetically various ingredients of our story. It is for this very reason that educated people in Western society, as they move through middle age, increasingly often turn to psychotherapy, or to some spiritual technique or cult, to pull the bits of their life together before it is too late. Sometimes this search for peace and harmony is not backward looking, but takes the form of living to the full the final stage as the fruit for which the tree was created—'the last of life for which the first was made'—but this is not so easy to do if your bodily functions are collapsing in an imprisoning or humiliating way. Others, again, never accept or become aware of the fact that their life is drawing to a close. They seem unable to see that there is nothing more the doctors can do, and talk as if they would eventually pull round and the story of their life continue for a further chapter. But these perhaps are not often found in hospices and so need not be discussed here.

The point I want to bring out is this. In various ways the kind of responses described all link value very closely with Time, and what has been done with Time. Moreover, they have a particular shape in common: a kind of self-contained curve. They are attempts either to give life completeness or to discern a reasonably satisfying completeness within it. Even behind the attitude of those who will not accept the approach of death, or for reasons connected with their clinical condition cannot take in the fact that it is approaching, there is a limitation of the horizon of concern to this physically based existence. 'So much to do' means that whatever is to be done has to be done within this scope. Paradoxically, this focusing on earthly time is found just as much in people who sincerely believe in a future life as in those who do not. The way we shape our span of Time in practice is not necessarily controlled by our religious or philosophical beliefs.

Nevertheless, there is another radically different kind of shape which can be given to life, and one that is organically related to belief in a future existence. Instead of being complete in itself it can be emphatically incomplete, a shape or pattern which demands something more to make sense of it, which is indeed designed with an eye to that something more. This is not at all the same as feeling unsatisfied with earthly life and with what has been achieved through it, or as wishing for that life to be extended. It is a characteristic of this different design that more of the same thing will not complete it. It needs something new in kind, if the purposes begun here are to come to fruition.

This future may be conceived in various ways. In Hindu or Buddhist thought it may be an escape from the wheel of *Karma* by which we are trapped in contingency, flux and suffering. In this future desired state individual personality, that which seems to the Western mind the most precious and essential of all possessions, will be dissolved, for it is precisely this clinging to individuality which is the root of desire and so of pain and subjection to the tyranny of death. The goal, therefore, must be a complete breaking free from the fundamental terms of life as we know it now. The wise or good person will, therefore, live this life in a way which will maximize the chance of escaping from the wheel of *Karma*, if not at the end of this incarnation, then after a series of progressively more virtuous lives. In Judaeo–Christian visions of existence beyond death the emphasis is very different. Though the thought of being 'lost in God' is not absent, especially in the mystical tradition, it is not the basic quality of the life to come. This is essentially one of individual fulfilment. That statement needs to be qualified. All branches of the Judaeo–Christian tradition recognize that there can be no satisfying or fulfilled life for the individual which is purely individualistic. There must be genuine and whole-hearted entering into relationships, not just that between the soul and God, but with other souls, as many and varied as possible. The individual must be a cell in a body, a partner in a huge and intricate dance, a receiver and transmitter of personal love. Nevertheless, despite this organic and corporate quality, perfect or eternal life is conceived as ultimately honouring and safeguarding the integrity of individual personality. The reason for this is at bottom a moral one, the deep conviction that any condition, to be morally worthwhile, must be free; and freedom requires an autonomous base for its exercise, even if that exercise is a constant surrender of autonomy. In crude terms, we may say that the antagonism between Oriental and Western religion or within Western religion itself towards the mystical tradition reduces to this: that the West cannot conceive of perfect happiness without independent identity, and the East cannot conceive of such happiness with it.

This contrast prompts two remarks. First that, because the tranquil acceptance of death demands a readiness to stop clinging on, to let literally everything go, to cease in any sense to act or to control the future, Western-type spirituality can actually make it more difficult to die. This has customarily been overcome in two ways: one, by teaching the believer to make his or her dying a supreme sacrifice or self-offering to God, in Christianity in union with the same sacrifice in Christ; two, by a depth of trust in the omnipotent, life-giving Creator which is convinced that God can and will re-create our being even beyond annihilation. There are other approaches, chiefly through some version of belief in the intrinsic immortality of the soul, but these two, used in concert, have been the classic means of coming to terms with death, where life after death is the controlling pattern.

These in their turn, however, call for supplementary assurances. Where God is thought of as upholding and eventually imposing a perfect moral order, belief that one's future depends totally on his goodwill can bring grave and distressing anxiety. Hence the central importance of the idea of the 'divine mercy', and the need to guarantee it by various means—atonement, sacraments, absolution, faith in the Word of God, and so forth. Since we are not perfect, our place in a happy future must be totally dependent on generous forgiveness by the One who is perfect, and who grants or withholds that future. In human terms, of course, this forgiveness, if truly believed in, is another and very effective way of helping the dying person to be at peace with their life, despite all its failures.

There is, however, a difficulty underlying every approach of this sort which theology has not until recently taken seriously enough, and which will immediately occur to anyone who works with the dying. It is the question: where is the essential person to be found? Even if we confine ourselves to the last hours of physical life there are problems. We all know how hard it is to be certain how much awareness or thought is going on, or what is the emotional state of the dying person. Those who can no longer communicate may, nevertheless, be conscious of a good deal; and this is one reason why physical contact is so important as the prime means of assuring them that they are loved and not alone. But over the inner life of the dying inevitably there is a veil that keeps much from our sight. In weakness and increasing isolation, how far are they still the 'same person' they were? Their identification is not in doubt—but what of their identity?

Taking this further, what do we say about a person's history? Nothing, it often seems to me, is more important for our psychological understanding of people than to be able to disentangle the permanent features of their personality from the genuine results of development. On the one hand, there are patterns of response, emotional dispositions, mental limitations and, running through all, a physical habitus, which remain recognizable throughout life. 'He was always the same, even as a child', we say; and in our own more honest introspective moments we recognize things about our public, maybe impressive, conduct which are just a new outworking of an old friend (or enemy!) within. We may be good specimens of ourselves or poor specimens; but we are still those selves, not some totally different self. On the other hand, there are facts about us which are equally real, equally part of us, but which do vary. Just as the same breed of rose may in one case be well shaped, strong in scent, glossy leaved, free from canker and so forth, or in another straggling, poor in colour, disfigured by disease, so may our personalities. And we can change dramatically from one period of our life to another. 'She's not what she was' we say, 'not at all the person I used to know'. The most drastic of such changes can, of course, be those induced by serious illness; and if the illness is terminal, it may be that, in terms of this life, the psychical deterioration is irreversible as well as the physical.

For any doctine of life after death the question must, therefore, arise: 'Which person?' Which is it that God re-creates, or which determines the next stage in the wheel of *Karma*: the person at the height of their power and virtues or the person crippled by adversity? On any assumption of justice (which underlies both beliefs) all ought certainly not to depend on what our forefathers called 'a good death'—something denied to the majority of human beings.

It has not been possible to do more than raise profound questions in sketchy and inadequate form. To conclude, however, I would like to try briefly to make two positive suggestions, which are a personal response to these problems. The first concerns the theoretical basis of life after death. The second tries to define one or two fundamental features in our relationships with the dying which are equally valid whether belief in a future life is present or not.

First, then, the theoretical basis. Unclear though my own thoughts still are, I am becoming steadily more certain that the only rationally coherent way in which we can think of future personal existence is in terms of *potential*. (Within the limits available I cannot, obviously, discuss such crucial issues as mind-brain identity, and so on, which are central to the plausibility of any doctrine of the kind; but since my concern is not to 'prove' a future life, but to unwrap some of the implications of belief in such a life, if it were true, I hope that what I am about to say can be illuminating even to those who do not share my own convictions.) By 'potential' I mean the kind of genetic analogy mentioned earlier: that is, the chance of becoming a 'good' specimen—indeed, as good a specimen as possible of the particular person we are. What goes to make up that person includes the personal history, perpetuated in two ways: the changes in characteristic responses and behaviour which the history has induced, and the memory of that history. To achieve the highest results of our potential we would have, in a future existence, both to mature in our responses and behaviour, and to integrate our memories positively and with love into a unified self. In theistic terms this means coming to see and rejoice in all that has been as an outworking of divine love—suffering love, no doubt, but as such the only way of overcoming the antinomies of evil.

It seems to me, therefore, that we need not be thrown by the 'which person?' problem, nor make dubious assumptions about God creaming us off as we were at some hypothetical best moment, or recreating an 'ideal' us. On the model of organic development (which is, after all, what 'life' means in our case) the whole story contributes to the future through the gift of memory, at present badly underdeveloped. Certain disabilities which arise from physical decay or weakness might well drop away after bodily death, and what the person had been speedily re-assert itself and go on from glory to glory.

One further point needs to be made. If a person is to have a good capacity for development in a future life, then clearly it is very necessary (as all religious traditions insist) that the spiritual, as opposed to the material, factors should be dominant here in this life. If someone has become more and more inert in this world, governed unwittingly by physical or emotional needs, never going against the stream of either inner compulsion or social convention, their personality in the human sense becomes less and less real. It could, indeed, very properly be said that the true objective of wise spiritual and moral training is precisely this: to make the personality more real, independently of its physical basis. It is no surprise at all, if we think about it, that those who have lived lives of intense spiritual and physical self-denial strike us often as far more 'real' and 'alive' than anyone else.

It is in those who possess this spiritual 'reality' that the idea that the line of this life is in fact incomplete, and demands to be continued in a much larger, perhaps infinite curve, strikes us as most convincing. But such people are relatively few. Our dealings are mostly with those in whom the pattern has no obvious shape, either for completion here or continuance hereafter. Let me end, then, with a brief reflection on one or two practical implications of what I have tried to say.

I remarked earlier that as human beings we link personal value very closely with Time, and what we have done with Time. If, then, we see the individual person not as a story coming to an end but as the beginning of an adventure leading to a unique fulfilment of glory, it can be easier, to say the least, to be positive about their value, to communicate to *them* an equally positive belief in their own value, to accept their failures and limitations, and to be glad for them even—sometimes especially—in the severest reductions of terminal illness. Moreover, for those who are linked with the dying only in the run-up to their deaths there must always be the artificial difficulty, perhaps suppressed from consciousness, of a limited 'professional' relationship. 'We are here just to help get you through this last bit.' One of the greatest achievements of the hospice movement is that it overcomes this built-in disadvantage over and over again by sheer personal caring. But I feel that an extra resource for overcoming it is available where either the dying person or the staff member or both can be aware of their relationship not as a more or less brief episode, but as in fact the beginning of a new enlargement in the pattern, which will now link both of them in love for the rest of their personal existence.

Belief in a new life ahead does nothing to question or invalidate traditional hospice methods, much less to suggest replacing them with utterly unacceptable pressurizing in the name of religion. It does, however, I believe, where it can be sincerely held, offer additional personal resources which both sustain the worker and can silently reinforce the supporting power of love to the dying themselves. The theological or philosophical reasons for tipping the balance of probability in the direction of belief in a personal future existence are, in their most valid forms, concerned with a moral question: does existence in the end say yes to value, that is, to goodness, truth, beauty, love? If so, then there must be something which is eternal in contrast to what we see all around us, including our own bodily life which is in flux and passes away. In traditional terminology, 'spirit' must triumph over 'matter', must make matter serve its own purposes. As we know, our bodies and the material universe around us are the vehicles of value for us. But when those vehicles pass away, does value endure? If it does, it can only happen through those sort of beings who understand value and can live by it. It may not be individual life in the very restricted sense in which that is understood in, say, Western European culture, but it must be personal life in some way. It is worth thinking about the meaning of that word 'person'—I know of no really more important question for religion, philosophy or ethics. If, as one suspects, it is in personhood that value has a foothold and is perpetuated, then for good to be eternal, persons must be eternal in some way or other.

We could never prove decisively whether this is the real state of affairs; one has to weigh the balance of probabilities. For the believers in various religions, the material of their beliefs is part of the evidence for their answer to that question.

Finally there is this matter of the shape of life. What do you do with Time? Do you understand your life as the business of making sense of your earthly chapter, coming to terms with it? That is one valid shape of the graph, curve or pattern of life. However, the survival, future existence or next chapter view does not presuppose a self-contained curve for this life. It sees this life as the beginning of something which may go off in most extraordinary directions. The equation for the whole curve is on that view quite unimaginable. It is not just a continuation of what has happened here; it is something different. For me, part of the mental conundrum is how to deal with both.

Meaning can be given to this life, but in doing that one need not close off the potential so that there is no point in thinking of another chapter. Surely one of the most fundamental things about people is that we are never satisfied. I suppose part of the poignancy of death for many people is the dissatisfaction. 'I could have been more . . .', 'perhaps we could . . .', 'perhaps we shouldn't . . .', 'I could have done more . . .'. At any rate even if I couldn't *be* more, there is more to experience, there are more relationships, more depths; the feeling of an unfinished story. That potential, I feel, must not be closed off; it is such an essential part of being human. And I feel sure it is what lies behind this sense of the future in the many diverse forms it takes in different religions and philosophies.

I find it very hard to assess whether the numbers of people who believe in such a future are declining in our society. Perhaps more people are ready than they were when I started work as a clergyman to say that they do not believe in anything—all sorts of religious taboos were still holding people back twenty, thirty, forty years ago. Whether this is so or not, there is a very important point with regard to hospice care: the relationship between the person caring and the person cared for takes on a different quality and meaning when there is openness to the future perspective. Whenever the doctrine of a future existence is shared between the patient and the persons caring for him or her, the concept underlying the relationship on the patient's side is: you are not doing this for only three weeks, three months, or whatever just to see me through this difficult passage, then writing it off and going on to another case. We are not like a lot of cars going through a garage for servicing or scrapping. Your care is the beginning of a personal relationship which will continue, and a friendship formed in terminal care is, in this perspective, a friendship which goes on. What you are doing for me is an enlargement of your experience; it is not just temporary or palliative. The people who support me at this moment are going to be my friends for life.

4
Current concepts of pain*

Ronald Melzack

The clinical phenomena of pain have often provided the basis for major advances in pain theory and research. Pain in cancer patients, for example, is determined primarily by pathological stimulation of tissues, but it is also profoundly influenced by psychological factors—the patient's past experience, religious beliefs, anxiety about the welfare of loved ones, anticipation of unending pain, depression about the prospect of death, and so forth (Saunders, 1967; Mount et al., 1976; Melzack et al., 1976). How does the central nervous system function to permit such powerful cognitive control over the somatic sensory input? Pain, it is generally acknowledged, is normally a signal that body tissues are injured; yet pain may persist for years after tissues have healed and damaged nerves have regenerated (Melzack, 1973). How can we account for neurophysiological processes that go on so long? Similarly, pain and trigger zones sometimes spread to distant, unrelated parts of the body. Can we understand such phenomena in terms of the known connections among neurons in the nervous system? While present-day physiology has answers to some of these problems, it is not even close to explaining others.

There have been significant advances in pain research and theory in recent years. The gate control theory (Melzack and Wall, 1965) has given rise to a massive amount of research in the attempt to reveal the mechanisms that subserve the modulation of pain signals in the spinal cord. Although there has been considerable controversy about specific details of the mechanisms, the concept of gating—or input modulation—is now firmly established (Wall, 1978). Physiological recordings from the cells of the substantia gelatinosa—the site at which gating is presumed to occur—have revealed a complex organization of excitatory and inhibitory influences from the periphery (Wall et al., 1979) and powerful descending inhibitory controls (Dubuisson and Wall, in press). There is substantial evidence, therefore, that pain signals are modified in the dorsal horns of the spinal cord before they are projected to the brain.

*Supported by grant from the Natural Sciences and Engineering Research Council of Canada.

Perceptual mechanisms

The time-course of pain is profoundly important in determining its psychological effects on an organism. Acute pain, which is usually associated with a well-defined cause (such as a burned finger or a sprained muscle), normally has a characteristic time-course and vanishes after healing has occurred. The pain usually has a rapid onset—the *phasic* component—and then a subsequent *tonic* component that persists for variable periods of time. Chronic pain states—such as low back pain, the neuralgias, or phantom limb pain—may begin as acute pain and pass through both the phasic and tonic stages. The tonic pain, however, may persist long after the injury has healed. It is then labelled as 'chronic pain' and appears to involve neural mechanisms that are far more complex than those of acute pain. The pain not only persists but may spread to adjacent or more distant body areas. It is resistant to surgical control and its prolonged time-course is characteristically associated with high levels of anxiety and depression.

Recognition of the difference between acute and chronic pain (Bonica, 1953) is now acknowledged as one of the major advances in the field of pain. In clinical practice, the relief of chronic pain requires procedures that are aimed at relieving anxiety and depression as well as procedures that modulate abnormal activity in the central nervous system (Melzack and Dennis, 1978). Before we examine these approaches, however, it is necessary to consider some recent evidence on conducting pathways and the nature of subjective pain experience.

Projection systems in the spinal cord

The fibres of the dorsal columns were long believed to carry information only about touch and proprioception. It is now known (see review by Dennis and Melzack, 1977) that they also convey information about pain by means of postsynaptic fibres that project to the dorsal column nuclei. The functions of these fibres are unknown, but it is reasonable to assume that they play a role in pain processes.

Dennis and Melzack (1977) have recently reviewed the literature on pain-signalling systems in the spinal cord, and found that six separate ascending systems (excluding the cerebellar projections) may have some role in pain processes. The six systems may be divided into two groups according to their physiological properties and anatomy.

The *lateral group* (Fig. 4.1) comprises the postsynaptic fibres of the dorsal columns, the spinocervical tract in the dorsolateral funiculus and the neospinothalamic tract in the ventral part of the spinal cord. Each of these systems carries impulses triggered by intense mechanical or thermal stimulation, as well as by innocuous tactile or thermal stimuli. Their axons tend to be well myelinated and conduct impulses rapidly to rostral relay cells, and thence to the nuclei of the lateral thalamus. The *medial group* (Fig. 4.2) comprises the paleospinothalamic and spinoreticular tracts in the

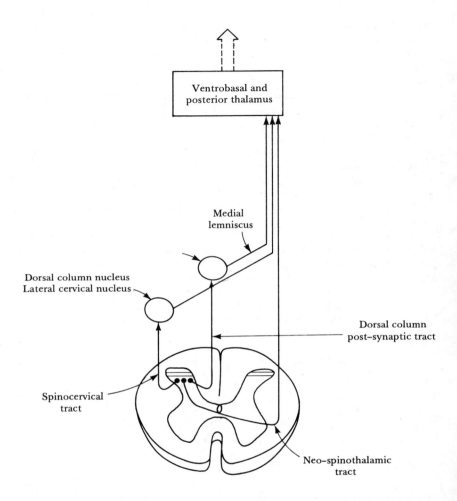

Fig. 4.1   The lateral pain-signalling systems. Three neural pathways arise in the dorsal horn of the spinal grey, particularly from laminae IV and/or V, and project rostrally across the midline. Each reportedly has elements that respond differentially to noxious stimuli. In carnivores, the dorsal cord pathways, particularly the spinocervical tract, appear to predominate. In primates, the neospinothalamic tract is pre-eminent. Impulses are carried by each system to overlapping regions of the lateral diencephalon, particularly to the ventrobasal and posterior complexes. A subsequent relay to cortex is likely. (Based on Dennis, S. G. and Melzack, R., 1979.)

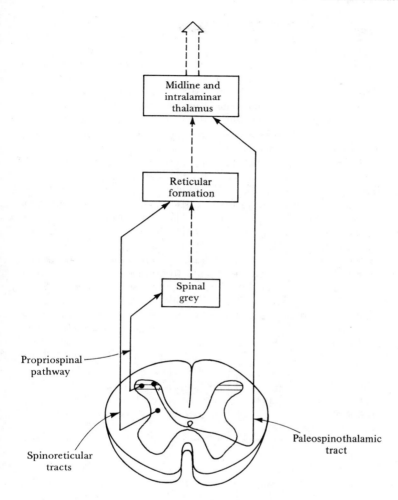

Fig. 4.2 The medial pain-signalling systems. Three neural systems arise primarily from the superficial and deep layers of the spinal grey. Each system should probably be considered as having bilateral projections, although only unilateral ones are shown. The propriospinal pathway depicted is only one of many possibilities throughout the cord. The rostral projections to the reticular formation tend to arise in the deep spinal laminae, and a number of different reticular regions receive fibres. The paleospinothalamic tract receives fibres from lamina I and projects to the medial diencephalon, in particular the nucleus centralis lateralis. The medial systems tend to maintain their relative sizes across vertebrate phylogeny. (Based on Dennis, S. G. and Melzack, R., 1979.)

ventral part of the cord, as well as the various propriospinal systems throughout the cord. The latter are less well defined, but are nonetheless implicated in pain-signalling. The systems of the medial group are multimodal, like the lateral group, but differ in other ways. These systems tend to conduct impulses more slowly. Perhaps most importantly, however, the information carried by these medial systems is distributed along the entire reticulated core of the neuraxis, from the spinal grey through the brainstem reticular formation, and into the midline thalamic nuclei.

Dennis and Melzack (1979) suggest that these two basic groups play specialized roles on the transmission of *phasic* and *tonic* pain-signalling functions. The properties of the lateral group seem to denote speed, security of transmission, and, via thalamocortical relays, rapid integration with all other sensory–motor processes. Such systems would be useful in transmitting phasic (transient) information, such as onset of stimulation or sudden changes in a noxious or potentially noxious stimulus. Responses triggered by such information would have adaptive value in minimizing the damage done by intense stimulation. The medial systems, on the other hand, are generally less rapidly conducting and synapses are frequent. Their target areas are less indicative of point-to-point relay of information than of global influences on information processing and behaviour. Such properties seem more consistent with tonic (continuous) information flow. There is less need for directness and speed if the message is to last for hours or days, as would be the case when tissue is damaged. Moreover, once damage is done, there is nothing the animal can do to escape it. Behaviour triggered by the message would be better directed toward preventing re-injury, resting and promoting healing. The possibility should also be considered that the medial systems, which play a major role in the affective–motivational dimension of pain (Melzack, 1973), directly stimulate the body's mechanisms for managing trauma, perhaps via hypothalamic mechanisms.

The measurement of pain

Recognition of the three major dimensions of pain—sensory, affective and evaluative—has led to a new approach to the measurement of pain experience (Melzack, 1975a). The measurement of pain in man is essential for the evaluation of methods to control pain. Yet the tools which are currently used encounter serious difficulties. Laboratory techniques for the production and measurement of pain have obvious ethical limitations on the intensity and duration of the pain that can be employed for experimental study. Laboratory pains are necessarily brief and are stopped when they reach unbearable intensity. Clinical pains, in contrast, are often persistent, unbearable, beyond the patient's control, and accompanied by high levels of anxiety. It is not surprising, therefore, that there are often marked differences in drug and placebo effects on clinical and experimental pains.

The McGill–Melzack Pain Questionnaire (Fig. 4.3) provides a new

McGill - Melzack Pain Questionnaire

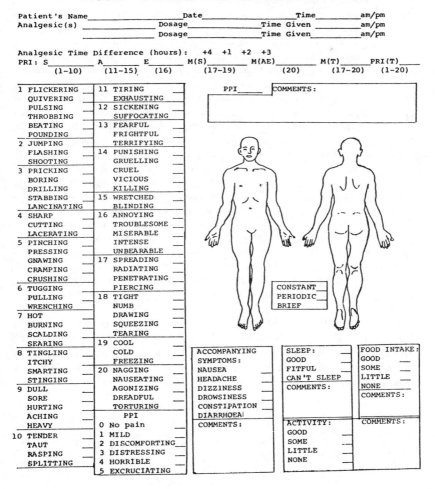

Patient's Name_____Date_____Time_____am/pm
Analgesic(s) _____Dosage_____Time Given _____am/pm
_____Dosage_____Time Given_____am/pm

Analgesic Time Difference (hours): +4 +1 +2 +3
PRI: S_____ A_____ E_____ M(S)_____ M(AE)_____ M(T)_____PRI(T)_____
     (1-10)   (11-15) (16)   (17-19)   (20)   (17-20)   (1-20)

1 FLICKERING ___	11 TIRING ___	PPI_____ COMMENTS:
QUIVERING ___	EXHAUSTING ___	
PULSING ___	12 SICKENING ___	
THROBBING ___	SUFFOCATING ___	
BEATING ___	13 FEARFUL ___	
POUNDING ___	FRIGHTFUL ___	
2 JUMPING ___	TERRIFYING ___	
FLASHING ___	14 PUNISHING ___	
SHOOTING ___	GRUELLING ___	
3 PRICKING ___	CRUEL ___	
BORING ___	VICIOUS ___	
DRILLING ___	KILLING ___	
STABBING ___	15 WRETCHED ___	
LANCINATING ___	BLINDING ___	
4 SHARP ___	16 ANNOYING ___	
CUTTING ___	TROUBLESOME ___	
LACERATING ___	MISERABLE ___	
5 PINCHING ___	INTENSE ___	
PRESSING ___	UNBEARABLE ___	
GNAWING ___	17 SPREADING ___	
CRAMPING ___	RADIATING ___	
CRUSHING ___	PENETRATING ___	
6 TUGGING ___	PIERCING ___	
PULLING ___	18 TIGHT ___	
WRENCHING ___	NUMB ___	CONSTANT___
7 HOT ___	DRAWING ___	PERIODIC___
BURNING ___	SQUEEZING ___	BRIEF___
SCALDING ___	TEARING ___	
SEARING ___	19 COOL ___	

8 TINGLING ___	COLD ___	ACCOMPANYING	SLEEP: ___	FOOD INTAKE:
ITCHY ___	FREEZING ___	SYMPTOMS:	GOOD ___	GOOD ___
SMARTING ___	20 NAGGING ___	NAUSEA ___	FITFUL ___	SOME ___
STINGING ___	NAUSEATING ___	HEADACHE ___	CAN'T SLEEP ___	LITTLE ___
9 DULL ___	AGONIZING ___	DIZZINESS ___	COMMENTS:	NONE ___
SORE ___	DREADFUL ___	DROWSINESS ___		COMMENTS:
HURTING ___	TORTURING ___	CONSTIPATION ___		
ACHING ___	PPI	DIARRHOEA ___		
HEAVY ___	0 No pain ___	COMMENTS:	ACTIVITY:	COMMENTS:
10 TENDER ___	1 MILD ___		GOOD ___	
TAUT ___	2 DISCOMFORTING___		SOME ___	
RASPING ___	3 DISTRESSING ___		LITTLE ___	
SPLITTING ___	4 HORRIBLE ___		NONE ___	
	5 EXCRUCIATING ___			

Fig. 4.3 McGill–Melzack Pain Questionnaire. Descriptors fall into four major groups: sensory, 1 to 10; affective, 11 to 15; evaluative, 16; and miscellaneous, 17 to 20. The rank value for each descriptor is based on its position in the word set. The sum of the rank values is the 'pain rating index' (PRI). The 'present pain intensity' (PPI) is based on a scale of 0 to 5.

technique to measure pain. The questionnaire (Melzack, 1975a) consists primarily of three major classes of word descriptors—sensory, affective and evaluative—that are used by patients to specify subjective pain experience. It also contains an intensity scale. The questionnaire was designed to provide quantitative measures of clinical pain that can be treated statistically. The two major measures that derive from the questionnaire are (1) the *Pain Rating Index*, based on numerical values that are assigned to each word descriptor, and (2) the *Present Pain Intensity* based on a 1–5 intensity scale. Correlation coefficients among these measures, together with experimental studies which utilized the questionnaire, indicate that the McGill–Melzack Pain Questionnaire provides reliable, valid information that can be treated statistically and is sufficiently sensitive to detect differences among different methods to relieve pain.

One of the most exciting features of the McGill–Melzack Pain Questionnaire is its potential value as a diagnostic technique (Dubuisson and Melzack, 1976). The questionnaire was administered to 95 patients suffering from one of eight known pain syndromes: metastatic carcinoma, post-herpetic neuralgia, phantom limb pain, toothache, degenerative disc disease, rheumatoid or osteoarthritis, labour pain and menstrual pain. In a multiple-group discriminant analysis of the questionnaire data, each type of pain was found to occupy a different region in the multidimensional space derived from the pain descriptions. Statistical analysis of the data revealed that the differences among the constellations of words for the eight syndromes are statistically significant. Each type of pain, therefore, appears to be characterized by a distinctive constellation of verbal descriptors. In a further study based on the discriminant analysis, the descriptor set for each patient was classified by the computer program into one of the eight diagnostic categories. A correct classification was made in 77 per cent of the cases. It is evident, then, that there are appreciable and quantifiable differences in the way various types of pain are described, and that patients with the same disease or pain syndrome tend to use remarkably similar words to communicate what they feel.

Modulating mechanisms

There are two major descending influences on pain-signalling pathways. The first comprises the brainstem system which is known to exert a powerful inhibitory effect on transmission through the dorsal horns of the spinal cord as well as other synaptic levels of the ascending systems. The second derives from the cortex and involves direct corticospinal tracts as well as indirect, multisynaptic pathways. Each of these influences is the basis for important new methods for the control of pain.

Hyperstimulation analgesia

There is convincing evidence (see Melzack, 1973 and 1975b) that brief, intense stimulation of trigger points by dry needling, intense cold, or injection of normal saline often produces prolonged relief of some forms of myofascial or visceral pain. This type of pain relief, which has been labelled (Melzack, 1973) as *hyperstimulation analgesia*, is one of the oldest methods used in folk-medicine for the control of pain. Interest in folk-medicine gained enormous impetus during the past decade by the rediscovery of the ancient Chinese practice of acupuncture—inserting needles into specific body sites and twirling them manually. More recently, the Chinese have practised electro-acupuncture, in which electrical pulses are passed through the needles. We now know that the original claims that acupuncture can routinely produce surgical analgesia have not been borne out by later investigation. However, acupuncture stimulation has recently been shown in several well-controlled studies to provide substantial relief of some forms of chronic pain (Co *et al.*, 1979). This is not surprising because it is now evident that there is nothing mysterious or magical about acupuncture; it is a form of hyperstimulation analgesia comparable to cupping or blistering the skin.

Transcutaneous electrical nerve stimulation has recently been found to provide a powerful technique for the control of pain (Melzack, 1975b). When it is administered the same way as acupuncture—for brief periods of time at moderate-to-high stimulation intensities (just below painful levels)—it frequently produces pain relief that outlasts the twenty-minute period of stimulation by several hours, occasionally for days or weeks. Daily stimulation carried out at home by the patient sometimes provides gradually increasing relief over periods of weeks or months.

A recent study (Fox and Melzack, 1976) compared the relative effectiveness of transcutaneous stimulation and acupuncture on low back pain. The results showed that both forms of stimulation at the same points produce substantial decreases in pain intensity but neither procedure is statistically more effective than the other. Most patients were relieved of pain for several hours, and some for one or more days.

In a related study (Melzack *et al.*, 1977), the correlation between trigger points and acupuncture points for pain was examined. The results of the analysis showed that every trigger point reported in the Western medical literature has a corresponding acupuncture point. Furthermore, there is a close correspondence (71 per cent) between the pain syndromes associated with the two kinds of points. This close correlation suggests that trigger points and acupuncture points for pain, though discovered independently and labelled differently, represent the same phenomenon and can be explained in terms of the same or similar underlying neural mechanisms.

Physiological basis of hyperstimulation analgesia
There are three major properties of hyperstimulation analgesia: (a) a moderate-to-intense sensory input is applied to the body to alleviate pain; (b) the sensory input is sometimes applied to a site distant from the site of pain; and (c) the sensory input, which is usually of brief duration (ranging from a few seconds to twenty or thirty minutes), may relieve chronic pain for days, weeks, sometimes permanently.

The relief of pain by brief, intense stimulation of distant trigger points (or acupuncture points) can be explained in terms of the gate control theory. The most plausible explanation seems to be that the brainstem areas which are known to exert a powerful inhibitory control over transmission in the pain-signalling system may be involved. These areas, which comprise a *central biasing mechanism* (Fig. 4.4), receive inputs from

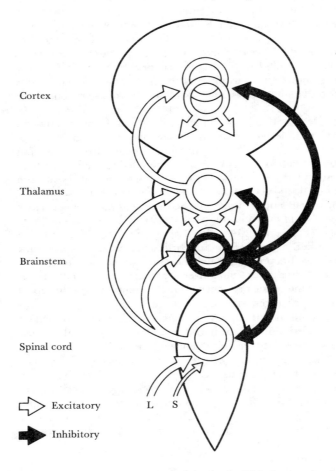

Cortex

Thalamus

Brainstem

Spinal cord

⇨ Excitatory   L   S

➤ Inhibitory

Fig. 4.4   Schematic diagram of the 'central biasing mechanism'. Large (L) and small (S) fibres from a limb activate a neuron pool in the spinal cord, which excites neuron pools at successively higher levels. The central biasing mechanism, represented by the inhibitory projection system that originates in the brainstem reticular formation, modulates activity at all levels. Loss of inputs to the system would weaken the inhibition. Increased sensory input or direct electrical stimulation would increase the inhibition.

widespread parts of the body and, in turn, project to widespread parts of the spinal cord and brain. The stimulation of particular nerves or tissues by intense transcutaneous electrical stimulation, or any other form of stimulation that activates a predominance of small fibres, could bring about an increased input to the central biasing mechanism, which would close the gates to inputs from selected body areas.

There has been recent support for this hypothesis. Direct electrical stimulation of the periaqueductal grey matter in the brainstem produces behavioural analgesia and inhibits the transmission of nerve impulses in dorsal horn cells that have been implicated in gate-control mechanisms (Oliveras *et al.*, 1974). Bilateral lesions of the dorsolateral spinal cord abolish these inhibitory effects and also abolish or reduce the analgesia produced by brainstem stimulation and morphine (Basbaum *et al.*, 1977). Furthermore, the analgesia-producing brainstem areas are known to be highly sensitive to morphine, and the effect of stimulation is partially reduced by administration of naloxone, an opiate antagonist (Akil *et al.*, 1976). The demonstration that naloxone also reduces the analgesic effects of transcutaneous electrical stimulation and acupuncture (Mayer et al. 1976; Sjolund and Eriksson, 1976) is consistent with the hypothesis that intense stimulation activates a neural feedback loop through the brainstem analgesia-producing areas. The analgesia-producing areas have also been found to contain endogenous morphine-like compounds (enkephalins and endorphins) and electro-acupuncture reportedly produces an increase in endorphins in cerebrospinal fluid in patients treated for chronic pain (Sjolund *et al.*, 1977).

The prolonged relief of pain after only brief stimulation requires the additional postulation of prolonged, reverberatory activity in neural circuits which may underlie 'memories' of earlier injury. These reverberatory circuits may be facilitated by low-level inputs, such as those from the pathological structures or processes that subserve trigger points or acupuncture points, and are disrupted for long periods of time (perhaps permanently) by a massive input produced by electrical or other intense stimulation. Furthermore, when pain is blocked, even briefly, the patient tends to become physically active and carry out normal motor activities such as walking and working. The normal, patterned proprioceptive inputs that result from these activities may prevent the resumption of the abnormal reverberatory neural activity that underlies prolonged pain.

Psychological modulation of pain

The problem of pain was long thought to be primarily the concern of the physiologist and anatomist, and the management of pain was almost exclusively the task of the neurosurgeon and neurologist. All this has changed in recent years. It is now firmly established that pain is profoundly influenced by psychological factors such as anxiety, suggestion, attention, prior conditioning, and a variety of personality variables. The problem of pain, therefore, has been investigated increasingly by psychologists, and psychological methods are, accordingly, often used in the treatment of chronic pain problems.

It is clear that new approaches to pain therapy are provided by recognition of the motivational and cognitive contributions to pain. Many of these psychological approaches are known to produce some measure of pain relief (Sternbach, 1978). They include (a) hypnotic suggestion techniques, (b) the use of conditioning procedures to diminish the frequency of pain-related behaviour patterns, (c) teaching patients to utilize feedback of electroencephalographic or other indices of physiological activity to develop a state of mind which allows them to cope with pain, (d) the use of stratagems to distract attention or change the meaning of the pain, (e) social modelling techniques, and (f) psychotherapeutic or pharmacological techniques to relieve depression. All of these approaches have value for the treatment of pain in some patients at least. They may not abolish pain entirely but may decrease some kinds of pain from unbearable to bearable levels for variable periods of time.

A recent review of the literature (Sternbach, 1978) reveals that a substantial amount of research is needed before it can be stated with certainty that any one of these methods is more effective than the others, or is more effective for one kind of pain than another. In fact, the widespread enthusiasm engendered by some of these new approaches is occasionally unwarranted. For example, there is excellent research on the effects of hypnosis on experimental pain but virtually no reliable evidence from controlled clinical studies to show that it is effective for any form of chronic pain. That hypnosis has helped many individual patients is beyond dispute, but it remains to be shown that hypnotic suggestion is any better than a placebo pill or sympathy from the family physician for the relief of chronic pain of pathological origin.

In contrast, there is convincing evidence that biofeedback therapy is effective for at least one kind of pain (Budzynski *et al.*, 1973). Tension headaches can be significantly reduced in about 65 per cent of people by teaching them to use muscle-tension feedback to relax the muscles of the forehead. The biofeedback training, moreover, was practised effectively by the patients in the home or office and continued to work in some cases that were followed for eighteen months.

Several studies have now shown that two or more psychological techniques used in combination often provide substantial relief of pain (Melzack and Perry, 1975). When EEG-alpha biofeedback was used in conjunction with hypnotic training instructions, the two procedures together produced significant relief of pain in patients with a wide spectrum of pain syndromes. Each procedure alone, however, failed to reduce pain by statistically significant levels. These results are not surprising. Pain is a multidimensional experience, involving sensory, affective and cognitive components. The effectiveness of psychological techniques—used alone, in combination with one another, or together with pharmalogical agents—makes them valuable tools in the fight against the debilitating effects of chronic pain.

The power of combined pharmacological and psychological effects has recently been demonstrated in a study of pain in terminally ill cancer patients (Melzack *et al.*, 1976). All patients received a solution of morphine (and a phenothiazine) which was taken orally every four hours. The dose of morphine was titrated for each patient in order to control the pain of the malignancy (Mount *et al.*, 1976; Melzack *et al.*, 1979). The 'control group' consisted of patients who received psychological and medical support from a multidisciplinary team in a special palliative care unit (PCU) in the hospital (Mount, 1976). The PCU was organized specifically to treat the symptoms and problems of terminally ill patients whose cancer was beyond cure. The purpose was to control pain and to provide comfort, care and attention to relieve as many of their anxieties and worries as possible. The results showed that the morphine solution produced significantly more pain relief in the patients in the PCU than in the other patients. Since the dosages of morphine and other drugs were comparable for the 'control' and 'experimental' groups, the significantly greater effectiveness of the morphine in the PCU can only be due to the psychological impact of the unit itself.

Central mechanisms

It is well known (see Melzack and Loeser, 1978) that about 5 to 10 per cent of paraplegic patients with total spinal cord transection report burning, shooting or cramping pains in parts of the body well below the level of the transection. There are many reports of paraplegic patients who had undergone removal of an entire section of the spinal cord (segmental cordectomy) in the attempt to alleviate phantom body pain, yet they still suffered severe pain in the denervated areas of the body. There is no reason to believe that the pain was due to depression or neurosis. Furthermore, the possibility that the pain was produced by nociceptive signals transmitted along the sympathetic chain is ruled out because the pain was not relieved by bilateral sympathetic blocks. Melzack and Loeser (1978) have described the following typical case history.

'W.B. sustained a fracture dislocation at D11–D12, with partial paraplegia, in an automobile accident. Immediately after the injury, a decompressive laminectomy was performed at D11–D12, and the surgeon noted that the spinal cord was contused and that there were several bone fragments within the dura. These were removed and the dura was repaired.

The patient complained of three types of severe pain one month after his injury. The first was a diffuse, burning pain perceived in his anesthetic distal legs. This pain was exacerbated by sitting and relieved by lying down. The second was a burning perirectal pain which was increased by anxiety or anger but was not related to position or bowel movements. A third pain was a burning sensation in his buttocks. This pain was particularly intense when the rectal pain was severe. W.B. was treated unsuccessfully with oral analgesics. Furthermore, multiple blocks of the peripheral nerves, lumbar subarachnoid space, and the lumbar sympathetic ganglia did not affect the pain. He was readmitted to the hospital 16 months after the injury and reported that his pain had not changed in the preceding year.

A spinal cordectomy at the D11 level was performed. Postoperatively the patient was noted to have anesthesia and paraplegia from the D11 level distally with no trace of sensory or motor function distal to this point. When seen 3-months postoperatively the patient reported that the spinal cordectomy had not altered his pain in any way. Although he did have intermittent relief of his burning rectal pain, this remained as much a problem as it had been pre-operatively. Sympathetic blocks did not alter his pain either prior to or after his cordectomy.'

Concept of a pattern-generating mechanism

On the basis of the clinical data, Melzack and Loeser (1978) have proposed that the loss of input to central structures after de-afferentation may play an important role in producing pain.

They suggest that neuron pools at many levels of the spinal cord or brain can act as 'pattern-generating mechanisms' (Fig. 4.5). These neuron pools are assumed to comprise the dorsal horns (i.e. the entire gate system) in the spinal cord. They propose that other nuclei along the course of the major somatosensory projection systems can also act as pattern-generating mechanisms. These cells are normally under sensory and downstream control. When de-afferentation occurs, however, the cells fire spontaneously in abnormal bursts for prolonged periods of time—a phenomenon that has been observed experimentally in several studies (Melzack and Loeser, 1978). It is reasonable to assume that the pattern-generating mechanisms, in paraplegics, must lie above the level of spinal transection or cordectomy. Furthermore, those regions responsible for pattern generation are assumed to project to the regions of the brain involved in precise localization of sensory inputs—that is, those neural areas that subserve the body schema—as well as to the areas that subserve pain experience.

The concept suggests that the prolonged bursting activity generated by the de-afferented neuron pools can be modulated by somatic, visceral and autonomic inputs as well as by inputs from neural mechanisms that underlie personality and emotional variables. Brainstem inhibitory areas are also assumed to modulate activity in the neuron pools. The loss of segmental input would lead to a decreased input to brainstem mechanisms that normally exert an inhibitory downstream influence on sensory transmission. The loss of descending inhibition would make it easier for non-noxious inputs to trigger the abnormal bursting patterns. Furthermore, the neural substrates of memories of prior pains, at spinal and supraspinal levels, may become active and also trigger abnormal firing patterns. The release from inhibition, moreover in addition to the sensory de-afferentation, would allow unchecked abnormal bursting activity so that the pain would persist for indefinitely long periods of time. The diminished inhibition would also allow recruitment of additional neurons into the abnormally firing pools and, thereby, underlie the intensification and spread of pain.

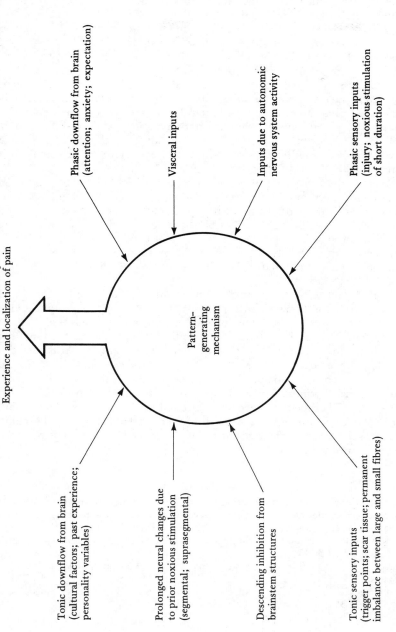

Fig. 4.5 Concept of a 'pattern generating mechanism' controlled by multiple inputs.

Implications of the concept

The concept of a central 'pattern-generating mechanism' (Melzack and Loeser, 1978) underscores central factors in pain and places peripheral contributions where they should be—at the periphery. There is no denying the role of neuromas, nerve injury, herniated intervertebral discs and so forth as major contributions to pain or as initiators of abnormal central processes. But once the abnormal central pattern-generating processes are underway, the peripheral contributions may assume less importance. They are, to be sure, avenues for modulating the activities in the pattern-generating mechanisms, but their removal may not stop pain once it is established. The proof of this statement lies in the countless patients who continue to suffer severe phantom limb, neuralgic and back pain after removal of neuromas, nerves and protruding discs, after extensive rhizotomies and multiple cordotomies, and even after total spinal cord transection.

Once the pattern-generating mechanisms become capable of producing patterns for pain, any input may act as a trigger. Thus, the emphasis for therapy lies in the modulation of inputs that affect the pattern-generating mechanisms. Decreasing the input by anaesthetic blocks or increasing it by electrical stimulation may be efficacious. Psychotherapeutic methods or drugs such as mood elevators and antidepressants may also be helpful. Aims and goals in life that make life worth living in spite of the pain may diminish both anxiety and pain.

The concept of central generating mechanisms which are triggered and modulated by multiple inputs has important therapeutic implications. Therapy at present is often predicated on a one cause–one effect relationship. In contrast, the concept indicates multiple interactions that determine the nature of the pattern which is generated. Attempts can therefore be made to change the pattern by *simultaneous* use of several procedures. Thus, it is plausible to provide patients with an antidepressant drug, electrical stimulation at trigger points *and* physiotherapy all at the same time. Therapeutic procedures in combination are sometimes more effective than the mere additive effects of each presented by itself. This kind of approach is reasonable in terms of central generating mechanisms as the cause of chronic pain.

References

Akil, H., Mayer, D. J. and Liebeskind, J. C. (1976). Antagonism of stimulation-produced analgesia by naloxone, a narcotic antagonist. *Science* **191**, 961.

Basbaum, A. I., Marley, N. E. J., O'Keefe, J. and Clanton, C. H. (1977). Reversal of morphine and stimulus-produced analgesia by subtotal spinal cord lesions. *Pain* **3**, 43.

Bonica, J. J. (1953). *The Management of Pain*. Lea and Febiger, Philadelphia.

Budzynski, T. H., Stoyva, J. M., Adler, C. S. and Mullaney, D. J. (1973). EMG biofeedback and tension headache: a controlled outcome study. *Psychosomatic Medicine* **35**, 484.

Co, L. L., Schmitz, T. H., Havdala, H., Reyes, A. and Westerman, M. P. (1979). Acupuncture: an elevation in the painful crises of sickle cell anemia. *Pain* 7, 181.

Dennis, S. G. and Melzack, R. (1977). Pain signalling systems in the dorsal and ventral spinal cord. *Pain* 4, 97.

Dennis, S. G. and Melzack, R. (1979). Comparison of phasic and tonic pain in animals. In *Advances in Pain Research and Therapy*, Vol. 3, Ed. by J. J. Bonica, J. C. Liebeskind and D. Albe-Fessard. Raven Press, New York.

Dubuisson, D. and Melzack, R. (1976). Classification of clinical pain descriptions by multiple group discriminant analysis. *Experimental Neurology* 51, 480.

Dubuisson, D. and Wall, P. (in press)

Fox, E. J. and Melzack, R. (1976). Transcutaneous electrical stimulation and acupuncture: comparison of treatment for low-back pain. *Pain* 2, 144.

Mayer, D. J., Price, D. D., Barber, J. and Rafii, A. (1976). Acupuncture analgesia: evidence for activation of a pain inhibitory system as a mechanism of action. In *Advances in Pain Research and Therapy*, Vol. 1, Ed. by J. J. Bonica and D. Albe-Fessard. Raven Press, New York.

Melzack, R. (1973). *The Puzzle of Pain*. Penguin, Harmondsworth.

Melzack, R. (1975a). The McGill Pain Questionnaire: major properties and scoring methods. *Pain* 1, 277.

Melzack, R. (1975b). Prolonged relief of pain by brief, intense transcutaneous electrical stimulation. *Pain* 1, 357.

Melzack, R. and Dennis, S. G. (1978). Neurophysiological foundations of pain. In *The Psychology of Pain*, Ed. by R. A. Sternbach. Raven Press, New York.

Melzack, R. and Loeser, J. D. (1978). Phantom body pain in paraplegics: evidence for a central "pattern generating mechanism". *Pain* 4, 195.

Melzack, R., Mount, B. M. and Gordon, J. M. (1979). The Brompton mixture versus morphine solution given orally: effects on pain. *Canadian Medical Association Journal* 120, 435.

Melzack, R., Ofiesh, J. G. and Mount, B. M. (1976). The Brompton mixture: effects on pain in cancer patients. *Canadian Medical Association Journal* 115, 125.

Melzack, R. and Perry, C. (1975). Self-regulation of pain: the use of alpha-feedback and hypnotic training for the control of chronic pain. *Experimental Neurology*, 46, 452.

Melzack, R., Stillwell, D. M. and Fox, E. J. (1977). Trigger points and acupuncture points for pain: correlations and implications. *Pain* 3, 3.

Melzack, R. and Wall, P. D. (1965). Pain mechanisms: a new theory. *Science* 150, 971.

Mount, B. M. (1976). The problem of caring for the dying in a general hospital: the palliative care unit as a possible solution. *Canadian Medical Association Journal* 115, 119.

Mount, B. M., Ajemian, I. and Scott, J. F. (1976). Use of the Brompton mixture in treating the chronic pain of malignant disease. *Canadian Medical Association Journal* 115, 122.

Oliveras, J. L., Besson, J. M., Guilbaud, G. and Liebeskind, J. C. (1974). Behavioural and electrophysiological evidence of pain inhibition from midbrain stimulation. *Experimental Brain Research* 20, 32.

Saunders, C. (1967). *The Management of Terminal Illness*. London Hospital Medical Publications.

Sjolund, B. and Eriksson, M. (1976). Electro-acupuncture and endogenous morphines. *Lancet* ii, 1085.

Sjolund, B., Terenius, L. and Eriksson, M. (1977). Increased cerebrospinal fluid levels of endorphins after electro-acupuncture. *Acta physiologica Scandinavica* **100**, 382.

Sternbach, R. A. (1978). *The Psychology of Pain*. Raven Press, New York.

Wall, P. D. (1978). The gate control theory of pain mechanisms: a re-examination and a re-statement. *Brain* **101**, 1.

Wall, P. D., Merrill, E. G. and Yaksh, T. L. (1979). Responses of single units in laminae 2 and 3 of cat spinal cord., *Brain Research* **160**, 245.

5
Symptom control in the dying patient

The principles of symptom control
Mary Baines

Thirteen years ago the first patients entered St Christopher's Hospice, and nine months later the writer joined Dame Cicely Saunders and Dame Albertine Winner as the third permanent member of the medical staff. During these thirteen years we have seen the principles of hospice care which Dr Saunders had enunciated work out in the community which is St Christopher's, and more recently in the hospices, home care teams and palliative care units which have sprung up in response to local needs throughout the world.

Hospice care has many facets, but excellent symptom control must surely be the first in importance. Unless it is present nothing else is possible. One cannot adequately help a man to come to accept his impending death if he remains in severe pain, one cannot give spiritual counsel to a woman who is persistently vomiting, or help a wife and children say their goodbyes to a father who is so drugged that he cannot respond.

For many years Friday has been 'Visitors' Day' at St Christopher's and the doctors are separated from the multidisciplinary group for an hour's ward round before lunch. Those who attend come from many parts of the world, work in different specialities and are of different generations, but four times out of five their motive in coming is to learn symptom control and they often talk of patients, past and present, with uncontrolled pain or sickness.

Every doctor or nurse has experienced a reluctance to visit a patient whom he feels he has failed and a pleasure in visiting one with whom he has succeeded. Only too often the dying patient is regarded as a failure. The hospice movement must give to doctors and nurses the tools they need, the ability to control pain and other distressing symptoms. Then they will again find satisfaction in caring for the dying and emotional and spiritual support for the whole family becomes possible.

The aim of medical training is to impart the ability to analyse past history, present symptoms, clinical examination and appropriate investigations in order to make a diagnosis. Most doctors will remember the thrill they had as a young house physician in diagnosing some obscure complaint in an emergency admission and having their inspired guess later confirmed; for successful diagnosis has always been one of the most satisfying aspects of medicine.

In our hospices we care for patients whose diagnoses have been made by others, but the skills we learnt as medical students must not be forgotten. We need to practise the same technique of analysis, but apply it to **symptoms**, not **diagnosis**. This is not for the hospice movement only; the many who come to our units need to be taught that symptom control is just as exacting a discipline as diagnosis and can be just as satisfying.

Perhaps the key to this approach is the regular and frequent use of the questions 'Why?' and 'What?'

'Why is this patient in pain?' 'Why is he vomiting?' 'What pathological condition at what anatomical site is causing this pain?' 'What biochemical disturbance could be making this patient vomit?'

We should, of course, ask these questions of ourselves and our medical colleagues. Also we should not be ashamed to ask the nurses and occasionally to ask the patient or his family. We must go on asking until the answer is clear and if necessary continue asking after death. At St Christopher's Hospice we have a post-mortem room and the invaluable support of Dr Richard Carter, who has been doing symptom-orientated limited autopsies over the last two years.

This principle of symptom analysis needs to be applied to all the symptoms which dying patients exhibit, but the two most commonly reported are pain and vomiting, and these will be examined in this paper.

In order to answer the question 'How does cancer cause pain?' an analysis was made of the cause of pain in the first 100 patients with malignant disease on admission to St Christopher's Hospice in 1980. The results are shown in Table 5.1. In no case was the cause thought to be purely psychogenic, though it was realized that depression and anxiety, family, financial and spiritual problems frequently lower the thresholds for pain and thus increase the total pain experience.

With such an analysis it is possible to attempt a rational treatment of cancer pain, treatment which does not simply involve the prescription of strong analgesics.

A suggested plan is outlined in Table 5.2. In this table the term 'steroid' refers to glucoccorticosteroids; 'low dose steroids' to prednisolone 15–30 mg daily or dexamethasone 2–4 mg daily; 'high dose steroids' to dexamethasone 8–16 mg daily. The dose should be gradually reduced when possible.

The ideal method of using such a table would be to apply the primary treatment for perhaps a week, in the expectation that the pain would be relieved or at any rate lessened and then, only if necessary, proceed to the secondary treatment.

Table 5.1 Causes of pain in 100 patients with malignant disease on admission to St Christopher's Hospice in 1980.

Patients with pain	82
Patients without pain	18
Visceral pain due to involvement of abdominal or pelvic organs (includes 7 with liver pain)	29
Bone pain	17
Soft tissue infiltration	10
Nerve compression	9
Secondary infection	6
Pleural pain	4
Colic, due to bowel obstruction	4
Lymphoedema	3
Headaches due to increased intracranial pressure	3
Pain in paralysed limb(s)	3
Generalized aches and pains	3
Non-malignant causes (includes bedsores (7), also constipation, piles, post-thoracotomy pain, indigestion, arthritis, corneal ulcer, gangrene)	17
Cause unknown	6
Separate causes of pain in 82 patients	114

However, we are often presented with patients in great distress, a long history of unrelieved pain and a short prognosis. In such cases it is indefensible not to use all available methods of relief. For example, Mrs K., aged 53, was seen at home on January 18th. She was known to have carcinoma of the breast with multiple bony metastases and she had previously had radiotherapy to her dorsolumbar spine and pelvis. She was complaining of very severe and continuous neck pain present for over two weeks. A clinical diagnosis of cervical spine metastases was made and she was started immediately on a combination of enteric-coated phenylbutazone 200 mg tds and morphine 10 mg four-hourly. The anti-inflammatory drug alone might well have been effective, but it only works in about 60 per cent of cases and this woman needed the certainty of immediate relief.

Fortunately, the combination was effective; on January 20th the report was 'more comfortable, a little sleepy', on 21st 'pain free on above regime'. Contact was then made with her Radiotherapy Department where she was seen on the 24th. X-rays showed almost complete disappearance of C4 and C5. She was fitted with a cervical collar and a course of five treatments was begun which was spread over two and a half weeks.

The dose of morphine was reduced and stopped on February 6th, the phenylbutazone tailed off over the next few weeks and in late March Mrs K. was told that she gradually could stop using her cervical collar. She remains at home, still pain free.

Table 5.2

Cause of pain	Primary treatment	Secondary treatment	To consider
Visceral from involvement of abdominal or pelvic organs	Analgesics	Low dose steroids may help	Coeliac axis block for abdominal pain; intrathecal block for pelvic pain
Bone pain			
Direct spread	1. Palliative radiotherapy 2. Non-steroidal anti-inflammatory drugs 3. Immobilization cervical collar pinning	Analgesics	Nerve block; low dose steroids may help
Distant metastases			
Soft tissue infiltration	Analgesics	Low dose steroids may help	Nerve block
Nerve compression	Analgesics	High dose steroids	Nerve block
Secondary infection			
1. Deep	1. Systemic antibiotics including metronidazole if possibility of anaerobes; local surgery		Nerve block
2. Superficial	2. Systemic antibiotics; local applications, e.g. povidone-iodine	Analgesics	Topical local anaesthetics
Pleural pain	Antibiotics if appropriate	Analgesics	Intercostal block
Colic due to bowel obstruction	Faecal softeners; antispasmodics, e.g. Lomotil	Analgesics	—
Lymphoedema	Intermittent positive pressure machine	Analgesics	High dose steroids may help; diuretics rarely do
Headaches from raised intracranial pressure	High dose steroids; raise head of bed	Avoid opiate analgesics if possible	Diuretics may help
Pain in paralysed limb(s)	Physiotherapy and regular movement of limb(s) by nurses	Non-steroidal anti-inflammatory drugs	Muscle relaxants

Although pain is the symptom most feared by patients and families suffering from cancer, it is probably not the most difficult to control—opinions differ as to which symptom is so, but certainly nausea and vomiting come high up on any list.

Before attempting to analyse the symptoms we should understand the mechanism.

In practice we have found at St Christopher's that anti-emetics have a wider range of action than Table 5.6 would imply. For example, a phenothiazine drug often appears to help vomiting from a cerebral tumour or a low obstruction. This is probably due to the fact that although the main effect of the drug is on the **chemoreceptor trigger zone**, there is a lesser effect on the **integrative vomiting centre** (Table 5.3). In vomiting which is difficult to control, experience has shown that a combination of anti-emetics acting at different sites in the vomiting pathway prove effective when a single agent has failed.

Table 5.3 The integrative vomiting centres in the midbrain can be stimulated in these four ways, as shown. During the act of vomiting the glottis closes, the soft palate rises and the abdominal muscles contract, thus expelling the stomach contents. During the sensation of nausea the stomach relaxes and there is reverse peristalsis in the duodenum. Anti-emetic drugs act at different sites in these pathways (see Table 5.4).

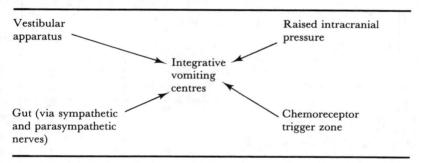

Other symptoms must be analysed in a similar way to attempt to find the cause, which may prove to be an anatomical abnormality, a malfunctioning or a biochemical disturbance. Thus treatment can be aimed at righting the wrong, or if this is not possible, the most appropriate drug chosen to relieve the symptom. Most symptoms require this sort of analysis: dyspnoea, cough, constipation and diarrhoea are some examples.

For the sake of simplicity, only the symptoms on admission of 100 patients were studied for this paper (Table 5.4). But patients dying of malignant disease continue to produce a multiplicity of symptoms, often referable to the malfunctioning of many systems. Good terminal care involves attention to all these and the doctor often feels like a juggler with new balls constantly being thrown in, attempting at the same time to keep the original three or four in the air.

Table 5.4

Group	Examples	Site of action
Phenothiazines	Chlorpromazine Prochlorperazine Perphenazine	Chemoreceptor trigger zone
Butyrophenones	Haloperidol	Chemoreceptor trigger zone
Antihistamines	Cyclizine Promethazine	Integrative vomiting centre
Metoclopramide	Metoclopramide	Chemoreceptor trigger zone; upper gut. Increases gastric peristalsis, relaxes pyloric antrum
Anticholinergic drugs	Hyoscine centre	Integrative vomiting centre

An analysis was made of any causes of vomiting in the first 100 patients admitted to St Christopher's in 1980. 65 patients were found to have no problem with nausea or vomiting. Table 5.5 shows the results of the analysis in the 35 patients with a vomiting problem.

Table 5.5 Postulated causes of nausea and vomiting in 35 patients (some duplication). In no case was the cause thought to be purely psychogenic, but as with pain, it was acknowledged that anxiety could worsen the symptom. Having studied the causes it became possible to offer rational treatment.

Obstruction
Oesophageal	3
High (pylorus, duodenum, jejunum)	2
Low (ileum, large bowel)	5
Constipation	1
Gross ascites	1

Biochemical changes
Hypercalcaemia	5
Liver failure	5
Uraemia	3

Gastric irritation, including gastric bleeding	6
Raised intracranial pressure	3
Drugs	1
With coughing	1
Cause unknown	6

This type of work must involve a fairly high level of medical staffing as a patient's progress needs reviewing daily at the start; later when things are under control it may be possible to drop this to two or three times a week. Symptom-orientated notes should be written so that progress can be followed. The nursing staff should be deeply involved, as the fine titration of drugs, particularly for pain, will often be done by them earlier in the ward or at home visits.

The doctor has a responsibility to keep up to date with advances in all fields of medicine, there are very few specialities which do not impinge on terminal care, obstetrics and sports injuries being the only ones which spring to mind! The doctor must be familiar with new drugs, although probably slow to use them. Hospices are not the right setting for trying new drugs, for so much depends on the confidence the staff have in the drugs they use. 'I'm so glad you've got that pill for sickness, I've found it works well' from a nursing auxiliary is invaluable. When new drugs are tried the doctor should, whenever possible, give an explanation of their value to the ward team.

The hospice doctor should have study leave, with time to visit other hospitals involved in caring for cancer patients; a week working in a radiotherapy department, a pain clinic or an active chemotherapy unit is invaluable.

At St Christopher's Hospice we have a recorder, Dr Joan Haram, who makes summaries of each patient's notes and from these annual statistics are produced. These cover not only the numbers of admissions, discharges and deaths, but also symptoms on admission, medication, insight and degree of symptom control. In spite of a widespread impression that the hospice is now admitting more 'problem patients' than at the beginning, the incidence of pain recorded as 'difficult to control' has steadily fallen from 7 out of 480 admissions in 1972 to 2 out of 591 in 1977 and 4 out of 626 in 1978. This is only part of the evidence for the success of symptom control based on the analysis of symptoms. The use of analgesic injections simply to control pain is now extremely rare, with perhaps one or two cases a year. The discharge rate has steadily increased and in 1978 was 12.5 per cent—social problems rather than uncontrolled symptoms prevented it from being much higher. Visitors to the hospice are often amazed at the alertness and cheerfulness of the patients, frequently openly disbelieving that the median length of stay is only twelve days.

Looking back at the early statistics one is perhaps surprised at the excellent results obtained at that time, far better than those found in most general hospitals then, or one must admit even now, in spite of the great volume of teaching from the hospice movement in the intervening ten years. At that time the drugs used were aspirin and other mild analgesics, diamorphine for more severe pain, and the phenothiazine drugs as anti-emetics and tranquillizers (Saunders, 1967). We used steroids to improve appetite, but we rarely used the anti-inflammatory drugs in bone pain and we rarely referred patients for radiotherapy. Those who have recently joined hospice teams will wonder how ever we managed.

Table 5.6

Cause		Primary treatment	Role and type of anti-emetics
Obstruction	Oesophageal—due to carcinoma of oesophagus or enlarged mediastinal glands	Radiotherapy; insertion of oesophageal tube	No use
	High—pylorus or duodenum	Consider NG tube; steroids occasionally help	Metoclopramide may help
	Low—ileum or large bowel	Faecal softeners	Anti-emetics acting on vomiting centre
	Constipation	Enema; suppositories; aperients	Should not be needed
	Gross ascites	Paracentesis with/without cytotoxic drug; diuretics may help	Anti-emetics acting on vomiting centre
Biochemical changes	Hypercalcaemia	Steroids: may need injection at first; use low maintenance steroids or eff. phosphate	Anti-emetics acting on CTZ* or vomiting centre
	Liver failure Uraemia	Do not modify diet; steroids occasionally help	Anti-emetics acting on CTZ* or vomiting centre
Gastric irritation	Carcinoma of stomach Peptic ulcer	Cimetidine	Anti-emetics acting on gut or vomiting centre
Raised intracranial pressure	Cerebral tumour	High-dose steroids; raise head of bed; diuretics occasionally help	Anti-emetics acting on vomiting centre
Drugs	Opiates, cytotoxic drugs, digoxin	Stop the drug	Anti-emetics acting on CTZ* or vomiting centre
Anxiety		Emotional support; tranquillizers	

*CTZ, chemoreceptor trigger zone.

What was revolutionary at that time was the regular giving of drugs to prevent symptoms and the titration of drugs against a patient's need—two of the great principles of terminal care first outlined by Dr Saunders. These have remained unchanged and are built into the framework of the hospice movement. It was these early years which revolutionized the care of the dying and inspired the opening of hospices and home care teams in this country and throughout the world.

We are more sophisticated now, more scientific, and quite rightly so. But never let us forget that our prime duty in caring for the dying is to give relief even if we do not understand the pathology. Patients must not be allowed to suffer while we undertake lengthy investigations or wait to discuss matters fully with colleagues.

By all means let us analyse the symptom as far as we can, be familiar with new drugs and techniques, but do not let us be surprised or ashamed if quite often we have to say, 'I don't understand what is happening, why he is in pain, why she is being sick, but I am going to try to stop it'.

The greatest principle of symptom control must be 'Get moving, and do it!'

Reference

Saunders C. (1967). The Management of Terminal Disease *Hospital Medical Publications Ltd.* London.

Therapeutics in advanced cancer: research findings

T. D. Walsh

Pain mechanisms

Neurotransmitters

Evolution in our concepts of pain mechanisms has been accompanied by an increase in knowledge of brain biochemistry. There are around thirty known chemicals in the brain which may function as neurotransmitters (Iversen, 1979). In pain pathways the role of serotonin (5-HT) is best established: briefly, manipulations which increase the availability of 5-HT potentiate analgesia and those which reduce 5-HT will antagonize it (Sternbach *et al.*, 1976). Morphine analgesia is affected in a similar fashion. The role of other monoamine neurotransmitters (dopamine and noradrenaline) and the interaction between them and serotonin is less well defined; dopamine is present in structures connecting the brainstem and forebrain, implying a complex role. Involvement of monoamines in pain mechanisms is of interest as they are thought to be important (Shaw, 1973) in endogenous depression. Drugs used in psychiatric illness which change monoamine function (tricyclic antidepressants and phenothiazines) are helpful in treating chronic pain (Kocher, 1976). There is good evidence for involvement of substance P in pain pathways, and presumptive evidence for somatostatin, neurotensin, angiotensin II and cholecystokinin. The topic has been recently reviewed by Sweet (1980).

Stimulation-produced analgesia (SPA)

Reynolds in 1969 showed that electrical stimulation of certain areas in the grey matter of the central nervous system produced analgesia. This SPA is extremely potent and outlasts the period of stimulation. Monoamine neurotransmitters are involved in both SPA (Akil and Lieberskind, 1975) and morphine analgesia. Increased and decreased (Akil and Mayer, 1972) availablility of 5-HT will promote and reduce SPA respectively. Dopamine depletion/blockade or increased levels of noradrenaline will reduce SPA (Akil and Lieberskind, 1975). In the mesencephalic periaqueductal grey matter of rats SPA is potentiated by increased levels of dopamine. Brain areas where electrical stimulation produces analgesia broadly correspond with the now known distribution of opiate receptors, e.g. periventricular grey matter (Pasternak, 1980).

Opiate receptors

In 1973 a number of workers demonstrated an opioid receptor in mammalian brain using radio-active naloxone (Pert and Sugden, 1973). Naloxone is a specific opiate antagonist used to treat opiate overdose. The technique was based on previous work involving insulin and cholinergic receptors. Martin and colleagues (1976) noted variations in the symptoms

Table 5.7 Opiate receptors (Martin, 1976)

Receptor	Agonist	Pharmacological role
μ	Morphine	Supraspinal analgesia, euphoria, morphine-type physical dependence
K	Ketocyclazocine	Spinal analgesia, sedation, anaesthesia, cyclazocine-type physical dependence
δ	N-allylnormet-azocine	Mydriasis, dysphoria, respiratory stimulation

and signs produced by different opiates both during administration and following withdrawal. This led them to propose the concept of multiple opiate receptors (Table 5.7; Gilbert and Martin, 1976). Cross-tolerance was demonstrated between morphine analgesia and SPA, thus implying a common underlying mechanism. Demonstration of the opiate receptor was followed by the discovery of the endorphin system (Hughes *et al.* in 1975).

Endorphins

The endorphins are endogenous brain opioids. The system comprises two components—beta-endorphin in pituitary and enkephalins in brain and spinal cord. Administration of both groups of compounds can produce analgesia (Goley *et al.*, 1979). Enkephalins interact with high affinity with a fourth (δ) receptor present in brain and mouse vas deferens. Morphine has low affinity for this receptor. Patients with chronic somatic pain states have low cerebrospinal fluid endorphin content; cerebrospinal fluid levels increase during opiate withdrawal in addicts, after acupuncture and SPA (Meyerson *et al.*, 1977). Analgesic effects of beta-endorphin and enkephalins are reversible by naloxone. Discovery of the endorphin system has been a potent stimulus to research.

Endorphins and tumours
Pullan *et al.* (1980) have demonstrated beta-endorphin and methionine-enkephalin production by malignant tumours and suggest endorphins are responsible for some physical and psychological syndromes associated with malignancy.

D-phenylalanine
This is a modification of the naturally occurring amino acid and inhibits a carboxy-peptidase responsible for enkephalin metabolism. It is reported to be analgesic in uncontrolled human studies (Ehrenpreis, 1978). Analgesic benefit can extend up to thirty days following one or two days treatment. No sedation, tolerance or withdrawal syndrome has been noted. In animals reversal of analgesia follows administration of naloxone but without production of a withdrawal syndrome.

Schizophrenia
There may be an abnormality of endorphin metabolism associated with schizophrenia (Torrey *et al.*, 1979). Psychotropic drugs are used to treat schizophrenic and chronic pain states.

(a) Pain insensitivity has been noted in schizophrenic patients (Torrey *et al.*, 1979).

(b) Naloxone is reported to reduce auditory hallucinations in some schizophrenic patients (Gunne *et al.*, 1977).

(c) Beta-endorphin injected intraventricularly in animals can induce catatonia, sometimes a feature of schizophrenia (Jacquet and Marks, 1976).

(d) Increased beta-endorphin and enkephalin levels have been described in cerebrospinal fluid of schizophrenics (Lindstrom *et al.*, 1978; Domschle *et al.*, 1979).

Narcotic agonist and antagonist drugs

The concept of multiple opiate receptors stimulated the search for more specific analgesic drugs. New analgesics were developed in the hope of separating analgesic actions from those considered less desirable, such as dependence or respiratory depression. Fundamental to this approach was the observation that signs and symptoms produced by cyclazocine and nalorphine differ from those of morphine. This led to the pharmacological investigation which is the basis of our current classification of the narcotic agonist and antagonist drugs (Houde, 1979).

(a) Pure agonists, e.g. morphine, methadone.

(b) Pure antagonists, e.g. naloxone, naltrexone. They have affinity but no activity at any of the proposed receptors. They oppose the actions of narcotic agonist and agonist/antagonist drugs and also produce withdrawal symptoms in patients dependent on these drugs.

(c) Agonist/antagonist analgesics, e.g. nalorphine, pentazocine, nalbuphine, butorphanol. Relative agonist and antagonist potencies vary. Characteristically, they are associated with dysphoria and psychotomimetic effects. They can produce an abstinence syndrome in morphine-dependent subjects, but cannot themselves suppress the morphine-withdrawal syndrome following withdrawal of high-dose morphine.

(d) Partial agonists, e.g. profadol, propiram and buprenorphine. Their actions are similar to morphine but limited by a plateau effect as the dose is increased. Psychotomimetic side-effects are not associated with these drugs. Large doses of partial agonists may precipitate an abstinence syndrome in opiate-dependent subjects.

There is little difference between the agonist/antagonist drugs and partial agonists in analgesic efficacy. Classification is complicated by variations in nomenclature and that above is likely to undergo further modification in the near future.

Anti-emetics: delta-nine-tetrahydrocannabinol

Vomiting is a common problem in advanced cancer and frequently inhibits optimal chemotherapy or radiotherapy during treatment of early cancer. There has been recent interest in the anti-emetic properties of delta-nine-tetrahydrocannabinol (THC), which is the component of marijuana responsible for its physical and psychological effects. Research was prompted by an open study conducted by Sallan *et al.* (1975) at Harvard which showed anti-emetic benefit when THC was compared to placebo. The same author has recently reported a controlled study of THC versus prochlorperazine (PCPZ) in chemotherapy patients who did not benefit from standard anti-emetic treatment. This showed THC to be superior to PCPZ. Chang and his colleagues at the National Institutes of Health in 1979 reported THC to be superior to placebo, a finding confirmed by Frytak's group (1979) at the Mayo Clinic, although the latter did not demonstrate superiority to PCPZ. Nabilone, a synthetic cannabinoid, proved to be a good anti-emetic in other clinical studies but was withdrawn because of toxicity during chronic animal testing. The increased appetite noted in some THC studies would be a useful bonus in advanced cancer. Studies reported are all short term and comparisons are difficult because of varying methodologies, although more general conclusions are possible (Table 5.8).

Table 5.8 THC—the story so far

An effective anti-emetic which is superior to placebo

Absorption is unreliable after oral administration (inhalation better)

THC blood levels may be related to the therapeutic effect

Euphoriant effect may be a prerequisite for the anti-emetic action

The commonest unwanted effect is sedation

Tolerance occurs to the anti-emetic action

THC may stimulate appetite and food intake

Relative efficacy to prochlorperazine requires further study

Nutrition

Nutritional supplements

The nutritional status of patients undergoing active cancer treatment has received attention in recent years. The reasons for this are summarized in Table 5.9. Anorexia (perhaps made worse by altered taste sensation) is a major problem. Nutritional supplements are of benefit during active treatment of cancer (Copeland and Dudick, 1978) and questions have inevitably arisen about their possible role in advanced cancer. Two mechanisms are basic to malnutrition in advanced cancer—anorexia and catabolism. Both may coexist and be made worse by psychological factors, therapeutic intervention etc. Before nutritional supplementation can be recommended in this group of patients, subjective benefit must be demonstrated as quality of life takes precedence over prolongation of survival. Concern has been expressed that nutritional supplements may 'feed the cancer' with effects opposite to those intended (Murray and Murray, 1980).

Table 5.9 Nutritional aspects of cancer

Malnutrition impairs immunocompetence (Munson *et al.*, 1974): chronic protein deprivation affects cell-mediated immunity more than humoral

Malnutrition alters metabolism of chemotherapeutic drugs (Basu, 1974)

Pre-operative parenteral nutrition reduces postoperative complications (e.g. after proctocolectomy) and improves outcome

Malnutrition may be the result of treatment, e.g. methotrexate and folic acid deficiency, 5-fluorouracil and sprue-like syndrome, intestinal radiotherapy and malabsorption

Reduced serum vitamin A levels are found in carcinomas of nasopharynx, lung and gastrointestinal tract. It is an immuno-stimulant (Soukop and Calman, 1978)

Low serum vitamin C (ascorbic acid) levels are seen in many cancer patients (see below)

Coenzyme A levels are low in some cancer patients, implying impaired B-oxidation of fats*

Metabolic rate and energy expenditure may be increased*

Abnormal riboflavin and trace metal levels may be found (Soukop and Calman, 1979)

---

* These changes are seen in non-cachectic patients.

Ascorbic acid (vitamin C)

Attention has focused on ascorbic acid because of the claim by Cameron and Campbell in 1974 for a beneficial effect in advanced cancer based on an open study of high-dose vitamin C treatment. Both subjective benefit and prolongation of survival are claimed. Cameron and Baird (1973) reported analgesic benefit with rapid (5–7 days) problem-free discontinuation of opiate drugs with the same treatment regime. A randomized double-blind study by Creagan and colleagues from the Mayo Clinic (1979) has not confirmed these claims. They were unable to demonstrate any benefit in advanced cancer either in terms of symptoms or survival. Vitamin C will continue to be of interest because of its role in physiological functions relevant to cancer biology (Table 5.10), and the controversy which surrounded Creagan's findings. The subject has received wide publicity with resultant patient self-medication. The matter must be resolved by further controlled studies.

Table 5.10 Vitamin C and cancer biology

Vitamin C appears to concentrate in some malignant tissues (Moriarty *et al.*, 1977)

Low levels are seen in association with many tumours

Vitamin C enhances the immune response—low levels are associated with reduction in macrophage migration and neutrophil phagocytosis

Vitamin C has a role in the synthesis and storage of monoamine neurotransmitters, some of which are involved in pain mechanisms (Subramanian, 1977) (highest concentration of the vitamin is in brain and adrenal cortex)

Vitamin C deficiency impairs drug metabolism (Zannoni and Likans, 1976)

Deficiency impairs wound healing

Increased collagen formation is seen (in the absence of vitamin C deficiency) in wounds in patients given high-dose vitamin C

Regression of adenomas in familial polyposis coli has been reported in patients given vitamin C

New drug delivery methods

MTS-1 continus

This is a slow-release preparation of morphine sulphate now available in Britain. Leslie *et al.* (1980) claim sustained blood levels of morphine are achieved for up to twelve hours. If clinical efficacy is proven this would be a useful preparation in home and hospital care.

Patient-controlled analgesia

Patient control of oral or parenteral analgesic dosage and frequency of administration has been tried in a number of centres for acute and chronic pain. The system has been used at the Memorial Sloan-Kettering Hospital in the management of pain due to advanced malignancy and has been found to be valuable (Coyle, 1979).

Epidural analgesia

Small quantities of morphine, e.g. 2 mg injected into the epidural space, are claimed to produce long-lasting effective analgesia, free of side-effects

(Behar *et al.*, 1979). The injection technique is well established and I believe has application in a number of advanced cancer patients where rapid pain control is essential, particularly those with short life-expectancy.

Continuous intravenous administration

Portable motor-driven syringes are available for delivery of drugs. Such devices are commonly used in hospitals for insulin and heparin infusions. Church in Australia (1979) and Rutter in Britain (Rutter *et al.*, 1980) have reported favourably on the delivery of pethidine and morphine respectively by continuous infusion for postoperative pain. Opiate side-effects are not a problem, and the doses of analgesic required to give good pain relief are smaller than when other means of drug administration are employed.

The future

Delivery systems allowing analgesics to be given across the skin or mucous membrane seem likely. They are already in use for other drugs (Zaffaroni, 1978) and may be particularly applicable to new high-potency analgesics such as buprenorphine.

Current research: St Christopher's Hospice

This section is mainly concerned with preliminary results from a number of retrospective studies. The data reveal the severe problems experienced by younger patients of both sexes and women with carcinoma of the breast during their final illness. Clinical relevance is the *sine qua non* of research in advanced cancer. The study concerning morphine and respiratory function is an attempt to answer a particular clinical problem.

The major current research interest at St Christopher's Hospice is the role of tricyclic antidepressants in management of cancer pain. There are many anecdotal reports of analgesic benefit from these agents used alone and combined with opiates. A prospective controlled clinical study to examine this area begins this year.

The data which follow relate only to St Christopher's Hospice patients. The approach to pain control can be summarized as follows.

1. All medication given orally if possible.
2. Morphine in water is the standard analgesic.
3. Analgesic dosage is individualized and titrated against pain.
4. Diamorphine is used intramuscularly when oral medication is inappropriate.
5. Adjuvant therapy, e.g. corticosteroids, is used as indicated.
6. An anti-emetic is routinely given with each dose of opiate.

Tolerance and oral morphine

Opiate tolerance or dependence are not practical problems in the management of advanced cancer pain at St Christopher's. In so far as it is

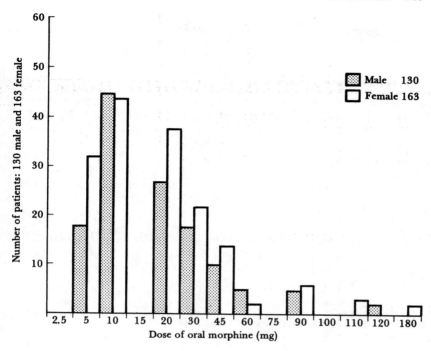

Fig. 5.1 Histogram: maximum individual dose of oral morphine, 1977. (Change from oral diamorphine to oral morphine 23rd May 1977.)

the only situation where long-term opiates are prescribed and this view is widespread amongst those in the field, it is surprisingly not reflected in standard pharmacological texts.

Examination of the maximum doses of oral morphine prescribed in the Hospice since 1977 (Figs. 5.1–5.4) makes it clear there is no progressive increase in morphine dosage; the majority of patients never go above the lower end of the known effective dosage range.

The final hours: problems and practice

This study examined the final hours of life in 200 consecutive patients at St Christopher's. We wished to define common problems and examine prescribing practices. In addition we were interested in any differences between patients who died shortly after admission and those who had been in the Hospice for some time. Commonest clinical problems were:
(a) respiratory distress;
(b) sedation;
(c) pain (on movement);
(d) agitation;

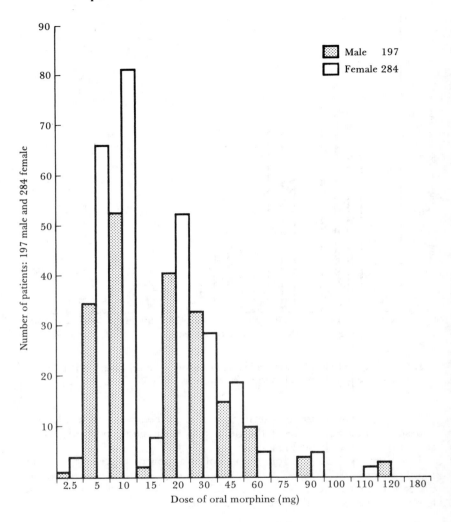

Fig. 5.2 Histogram: maximum individual dose of oral morphine, 1978.

in descending order of frequency (Table 5.11). Rank order is the same irrespective of age group or sex.

Young patients of either sex had more complex problems in comparison to the older age group. Nausea occurred exclusively and vomiting predominantly in females. Confusion was also more common in females.

Most patients were given diamorphine intramuscularly in the final

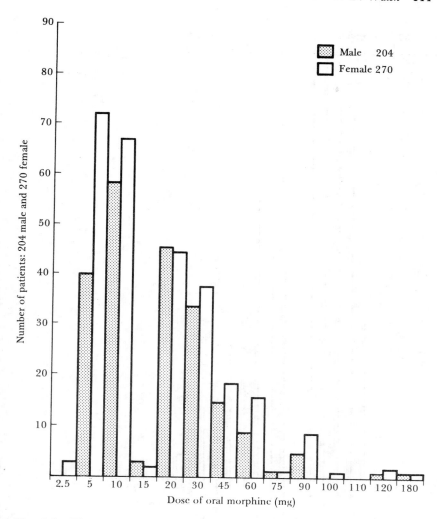

Fig. 5.3   Histogram: maximum individual dose of oral morphine, 1979.

24-hour period. Females (< 65 years) began diamorphine earlier than other patients (seventy-two or forty-eight hours before death): in contrast, elderly males tended to get diamorphine only in the last twenty-four hours. One-quarter of the patients did not get oral morphine at all in their final illness. Twenty-eight patients (14 per cent) got maintenance diamorphine before the last seventy-two hours—the majority females. The average length of this diamorphine treatment was six days, with younger patients

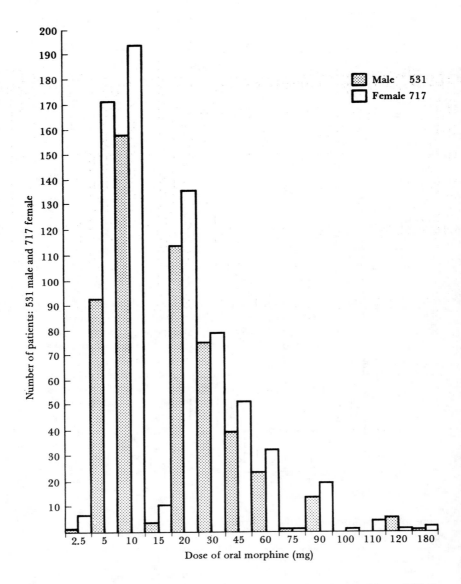

Fig. 5.4 Histogram: maximum individual dose of oral morphine, 1977–9. (Change from oral diamorphine to oral morphine 23rd May 1977.)

Table 5.11 Clinical problems of the last twenty-four hours in 200 consecutive patients 78/500 – 79/44

Age group	Female			Male			
	<65	>65	Total	<65	>65	Total	Grand
Total	45	75	120	27	53	80	total
'Chesty'	25	41	66	13	28	41	107
Drowsy	20	36	56	13	25	38	94
Agitation	16	20	36	11	16	27	63
Dyspnoea	13	15	28	10	15	25	53
Pain	14	12	26	8	13	21	47
Confusion	7	10	17	4	3	7	24
Twitching	2	8	10	2	4	6	16
Vomiting	5	7	12	1	1	2	14
Dysphagia	3	1	4	1	5	6	9
Nausea	5	1	6	—	—	—	6

getting higher doses. Vomiting was common in these patients (presumably the reason for parenteral treatment). The short duration of maintenance diamorphine treatment indicated end-stage illness with short prognosis. Chlorpromazine for sedation is given more often to elderly males and young females.

Examination of records of those patients dying within seventy-two hours of admission revealed no significant differences in clinical problems. Prescribing practice was very similar. Elderly males tended to die more quickly following admission (Tables 5.12 and 5.13).

Painful cancers: high-dose morphine patients

Analysis of Hospice records revealed 124 patients who got more than 20 mg oral morphine four-hourly in 1979 for chronic cancer pain. This high-dose morphine (HDM) group received one of the following doses four-hourly: 30, 45, 60, 90 or 120 mg. Data presented should be interpreted keeping in mind the lack of information concerning morphine pharmacokinetics.

There was an equal distribution of HDM patients between the sexes, although examination of the age distribution shows that members of both sexes under 65 years are more likely to get HDM. This trend is most pronounced in females. The male primary site involved was predominantly bronchus. Bronchial carcinoma comprises one-third of the total male primary sites of the year but half of the male HDM.

Carcinoma of the oesophagus, head and neck carcinomas and

Table 5.12 The final hours: 200 consecutive patients (1978–9)

Age group Total	Female <65 45	>65 75	Total 120	Male <65 27	>65 53	Total 80
IM diamorphine						
Last 24 hours	41 (91.11%)	66 (88.00%)	107 (89.16%)	24 (88.89%)	48 (90.57%)	72 (90.00%)
24–48 hours	21 (46.67%)	34 (45.33%)	55 (45.83%)	13 (48.15%)	18 (33.96%)	31 (38.75%)
48–72 hours	24 (53.33%)	24 (32.00%)	48 (40.00%)	11 (40.74%)	10 (18.87%)	21 (26.25%)
Last 24 hours only	17 (37.78%)	32 (42.67%)	49 (40.83%)	8 (29.63%)	28 (52.83%)	36 (45.00%)
Last 3 × 24 hours	15 (33.33%)	24 (32.00%)	39 (32.50%)	9 (33.33%)	8 (15.09%)	17 (21.25%)
Chlorpromazine						
Last 72 hours	32 (71.11%)	50 (66.69%)	82 (68.33%)	17 (62.76%)	46 (86.79%)	63 (78.75%)

Table 5.13 The final hours: 200 patients. Maintenance diamorphine (DM): patients on parenteral opiate **before** the final seventy-two hours. (Number of patients, 28 (14.00%); females, 21 (17.50%); males, 7 (8.75%); females <65, 8 >65, 13 ; males <65, 5 >65, 2

Age groups	Female 8<65	13>65	Total 21	Male 5<65	2>65	Total 7	Grand total 28
maintenance DM (days)							
Total	37	80	117	38	14	52	169
Mean	4.64	6.15	5.57	7.60	7	7.43	6.04
Mean initial dose DM (mg)	16.25	5.77	9.76	19	3.75	14.64	11.34
Mean highest dose DM (mg)	24.38	9.62	15.24	22	10	18.57	16.07

lymphomas are over-represented in males. A high proportion of each of these primary sites enters the high-dose morphine category. In females carcinomas of the cervix, and head and neck, as well as lymphomas and melanomas are present in the HDM group in excess (Tables 5.14 and 5.15). Group survival times from the first time that HDM was prescribed were similar. Overall length of illness was longer in females. Bone metastases were common (half of the men and a third of the women). Depression occurred more often in HDM patients of both sexes in comparison to the overall incidence in St Christopher's patients. Young women were most likely to be treated with antidepressants.

Table 5.14 High-dose morphine (HDM): primary sites (male). (Male total primary, 281; male total HDM, 59.)

Primary site	Common primary site HDM	Total primary site for year
Bronchus	29	100
Colon/rectum	6	32
Oesophagus	5	10
Head and neck	5	13
Prostate	4	22
Stomach	3	29
Lymphoma	2	2

Table 5.15 High-dose morphine (HDM): primary sites (female). (Female total primary, 364; female total HDM, 65.)

Primary site	Common primary site HDM	Total primary site for year
Breast	15	87
Colon/rectum	10	56
Cervix	9	19
Bronchus	8	41
Melanoma	5	11
Head and neck	4	8
Ovary	3	19
Lymphoma	2	3

Antidepressants in advanced cancer: two years experience (1977–1978)

Antidepressant prescribing was reviewed in preparation for a prospective study of the use of tricyclic antidepressants (TCAD) in *pain* due to advanced cancer. Only cancer patients given TCAD for *depression* were included in this study.

The majority of patients were women (Table 5.16). They predominated in both years' admission figures but were proportionately more common in TCAD group when difference in admission rates was considered. Dothiepin is the most commonly used drug. Amitriptyline, imipramine and trimipramine account for most of the remainder. The majority of patients received less than 75 mg per day and tended to get the same dose throughout their treatment, irrespective of starting dose.

The primary site distribution showed over-representation of breast, cervix, ovary and bladder when considered as a proportion of total

Table 5.16 Antidepressants (1977/8)

176 patients (14.46%)

Female : male ratio 2 : 1

Certain primary sites present in excess,
    e.g. breast, ovary, cervix, bladder

Excess primary sites associated with
    prolonged survival

Bony metastases common (25%)

Severe pain/high-dose morphine common
(>40%)

admissions for those primary sites for either year. Examination of survival by primary site revealed prolonged survival in TCAD group in relation to mean values for either year. Mean survival for 1977 and 1978 was 23 and 19 days respectively. Mean survival of TCAD patients was 32.47 days (1977) and 30.71 days (1978). Survival of over-represented primary sites was much longer, e.g. breast 70.31 days (1977) and 50.36 days (1978). Frequently, patients did not live long enough for TCAD to exert a therapeutic effect, but for those who got more than a week's treatment the mean duration of treatment exceeded four weeks. Clinical features of the illnesses in which TCAD are prescribed reveal some aspects of note. Severe pain was a common feature at some stage of the illness in nearly half the patients. More than a third received high-dose oral morphine (i.e. > 20 mg morphine four-hourly). Bony secondary lesions were common. Mean total length of illness was less than twenty-four months. Adjunctive therapy was prescribed frequently (e.g. phenothiazine, benzodiazepine), particularly for males. It is interesting that there is a strong association between use of corticosteroids and subsequent need for TCAD in men. The study suggests that depression could be the result of long-term opiate/phenothiazine treatment, although it may be solely a reflection of a long final illness.

Pain problems (1972–1978)

The study involved thirty-eight patients in whom pain control was a problem. Patients are selected yearly by the same experienced clinical studies department staff from summaries prepared by the Hospice Recorder, Dr B. J. Haram. Inclusion does not mean pain was uncontrollable but that difficulty was experienced in providing relief by usually effective methods. Data must be viewed in the light of increasing clinical experience and changes in clinical practice during the time-period discussed. Among the latter was the change-over from oral Brompton Mixture (diamorphine, alcohol and cocaine) to oral morphine in water (no diamorphine, alcohol or cocaine) in mid-1977.

Patients are fairly equally divided between sexes and by sex within age groups (over and under 65 years). In total there were 20 men and 18 women, but the age distribution shows the majority (31) of the patients are in the younger age-group (under 65 years). Male age range was 18–76 years, with a median of 53 years. Female age range was 32–71 years, with a median value of 54 years.

In women, carcinoma of the breast is commonest, particularly in those under 65 years (11 of 15 primary sites). There was a greater number of individual primary sites in males. Carcinoma of the bronchus (4) and colon (4) account for half of the male primary sites under 65 years (Table 5.17).

The clinical features show a pattern of severe complicated illness (Table 5.18). Metastatic bone disease was present in half the patients of both sexes. Amongst women with carcinoma of the breast, 8 of 15 patients had bony secondaries. Illness due to a primary site in a 'pelvic' organ accounted for

Table 5.17 Pain problems (1972 – 8); primary sites (primary sites total = 38)

Primary site	Age	Total	Primary site	Age	Total
Female	<65	15		>65	3
Breast		11	Stomach		2
Colon/rectum		2	Uterus		1
Bronchus		1			
Vulva		1			
Male	<65	16		>65	4
Bronchus		4	Bronchus		1
Colon		4	Pancreas		1
Prostate		1	Bladder		1
Pancreas		1	Prostate		1
Bladder		1			
Thymus		1			
Maxilla		1			
Testicle		1			
Sarcoma		1			
Unknown		1			

Table 5.18 Pain problems (1972 – 8): clinical features

Total patients	38
Male	20
Female	18
Metastases	
non-bony	32
bony	19
Anxiety	18
Antidepressant medication	17
Vomiting	14
'Pelvic' primary site	12
Patient insight	21

nearly a third of the patients. Clinical experience indicates that severe pain is often associated with carcinomas arising in this area (colon/rectum, bladder, prostate, cervix, uterus and ovary). Twenty-one patients knew their specific diagnosis but it is unclear if they understood the prognostic implications. Metastases in organs other than bone were very common, being present in 32 of the 38. Anxiety, vomiting and depression were next in descending order of frequency. Fifteen patients had antidepressants prescribed, but only 8 had diagnosis recorded. This probably reflects drugs begun for depression prior to admission.

Opiate prescribing showed that 17 men and 15 women got in excess of 20 mg morphine four-hourly (or its diamorphine eqivalent, based on an oral diamorphine : morphine potency ratio 1 : 1.5). There was no detectable difference between age groups in opiate prescribing.

Oral morphine and respiratory function in advanced cancer

One problem preventing optimal use of opiates for cancer pain is fear of respiratory depression causing premature death of the patient. An open prospective study of respiratory function in HDM group is in progress. All these patients get a minimum of 150 mg oral morphine per twenty-four

Table 5.19 Oral morphine/respiratory function study

Entry criteria
Breathing room air
Stable physical condition
Pain free
No acute chest/chest-wall disease
Examined sitting/lying after fifteen minutes rest
Morphine dose >20 mg four-hourly
Morphine prescribed for minimum of seven days, and at a stable dose for more than seventy-two hours

Table 5.20 Oral morphine/respiratory function study

Investigations
Clinical status
Pain ±
Respiratory rate
Peak flow
Blood
gases
urea
creatinine
electrolytes
morphine level (trough)

Peak flow readings unreliable because of poor patient co-operation; all investigations carried out at 'trough' of morphine plasma level.

hours. Oral morphine is prescribed in the Hospice in individualized doses titrated against the patient's pain. Entry criteria for the study are shown in Table 5.19, investigations in Table 5.20 and individual patient results (in thirteen patients examined so far) in Table 5.21. There is no evidence of ventilatory depression. The study is not complete, but results obtained are encouraging and support clinical experience. Morphine undoubtedly may cause respiratory depression, but we believe this is untrue in cancer patients where oral morphine dosage is titrated against pain. We are now proceeding to studies in patients receiving oral morphine for the first time.

Table 5.21 Oral morphine/respiratory function study

Age	Primary	Morphine dose (mg) four-hourly	Respiratory rate/min.	Peak flow	P_{CO_2}
Female					
45	Breast	30	12	300	39.6
48	Sigmoid colon	30	16	200	36.5
54	Gall bladder	60	12	240	38.5
54	Breast	30	16	240	36.3
Male					
45	Bronchus	30	12	350	29.5
48	Unknown	30	16	320	30.8
52	Bronchus	30/45	16	300	39.5
56	Prostate, stomach	30	20	100	40.3
58	Bladder	30	16	170	44.5
62	Stomach	30	16	320	40.9
74	Bronchus	30	22	330	40.6
75	Bronchus	45/60	16	220	41.7
79	Bronchus	30/20	18	120	25.8

References

Akil, H. and Lieberskind, J. C. (1975). Monoaminergic mechanisms of stimulation-produced analgesia. *Brain Research* **94**, 279.

Akil, H. and Mayer, D. J. (1972). Antagonism of stimulation-produced analgesia by p-CPA a serotonin synthesis inhibitor. *Brain Research* **44**, 692.

Basu, T. K. (1974). Inter-relationships of nutrition and the metabolism of drugs. *Chemical and Biological Interactions.* **8**, 193.

Behar, M., Olshwang, D., Margora, F. and Davidson, J. T. (1979). Epidural morphine in treatment of pain. *Lancet* **i**, 527.

Cameron, E. and Baird, G. M. (1973). Ascorbic acid and dependence on opiates in patients with advanced disseminated cancer. (Letter). Journal of Int. Res. Commun. **1**, 38.

Cameron, E. and Campbell, A. (1974). The orthomolecular treatment of cancer. II. Clinical Trial of High-dose Ascorbic Acid Supplements in Advanced Human Cancer. *Chemical and Biological Interactions* **9**, 285.

Chang, A. E., Shiling, D. J., Stillman, R. C. *et al.* (1979). Delta-9-tetrahydrocannabinol as an antiemetic in cancer patients receiving high-dose methotrexate. *Annals of Internal Medicine* **91**, 819.

Church, J. J. (1979). Continuous narcotic infusions for relief of postoperative pain. *British Medical Journal* **1**, 977.

Copeland, E. M. III. and Dudrick, S. J. (1978). The importance of parenteral nutrition as an adjunct to cancer treatment. In *Advances in Parenteral Nutrition*, Ed. by J. D. A. Johnston. M.T.P. Press, Lancaster.

Coyle, N. (1979). Analgesics at the bedside. *American Journal of Nursing* **9**, 1554.

Creagan, E. T., Moertel, C. G., O'Fallon, J. R. *et al.* (1979). Failure to high-dose vitamin C (ascorbic acid) therapy to benefit patients with advanced cancer. *New England Journal of Medicine* **301**, 687.

Domschle, W., Dickschas, A. and Mitzwegg, P. (1979). C. S. F. β-endorphin in schizophrenia. *Lancet* **i**, 1024.

Ehrenpreis, S. (1978). Once-a-month drug stops pain in preliminary trials. *Medical World News*, p.10.

Foley, K. M., Korindes, I. A., Inturrisi, C. E. *et al.* (1979). Beta-endorphin: analgesic and hormonal effects in humans. *Proceedings of the National Academy of Science (USA)* **76**, 1.

Frytak, S., Moertal, C. G., O'Fallon, J. R. *et al.* (1979). Delta-9-tetrahydrocannabinol as an antiemetic for patients receiving cancer themotherapy. *Annals of Internal Medicine* **91**, 825.

Gilbert, P. E. and Martin, W. R. (1976). The effects of morphine and nalorphine-like drugs in the non-dependent, morphine-dependent and cyclazocine-dependent chronic spinal dog. *Journal of Pharmacology and Experimental Therapeutics* **198**, 66.

Gunne, L. M., Lindstrom, L. and Terenius, L. (1977). Naloxone-induced reversal of schizophrenic hallucinations. *Journal of Neurotransmission* **40**, 13.

Houde, R. W. (1979). Analgesic effectiveness of the narcotic agonist–antagonists. *British Journal of Clinical Pharmacology* **7** (suppl. 3) 298S.

Hughes, J., Smith, T. W., Kosterlitz, H. W. *et al.* (1975). Identification of two related pentapeptides from the brain with potent opiate agonist activities. *Nature* **258**, 577.

Iversen, L. L. (1979). The chemistry of the brain. *Scientific American* **241**, 118.

Jacquet, Y. F. and Marks, N. (1976). The c-fragment of β-lipotropin: an endogenous neuroleptic or antipsychotogen. *Science* **194**, 632.

Kocher, R. (1976). The use of psychotropic drugs in the treatment of chronic, severe pains. *European Neurology* **14**, 458.

Kosterlitz, H. W., Collier, H. O. J. and Villareal, J. E. (Eds.) (1971). Receptor dualism: some kinetic implications in agonist and antagonist actions of narcotic analgesic drugs. *Proceedings of the Symposium of the British Pharmacological Society, July 1971.* Macmillan, London.

Leslie, S. T., Black, F. M., Boroda, C. and Rhodes, A. (1980). A controlled release morphine sulphate tablet—a study in normal volunteers. *British Journal of Clinical Pharmacology* **9**, 531

Lindstrom, L. H., Widerlov, E., Junne, L. M. *et al.* (1978). Endorphin in human cerebrospinal fluid: clinical correlation to some psychotic states. *Acta Psychiatrica Scandinavia* **57**, 153.

Meyerson, B. J., Boethius, J., Terenins, L. and Wahlstrom, A. (1977). Endorphin mechanisms in pain relief with intracerebral and dorsal column stimulation. 3rd Meeting of the European Society of Stereotactic and Functional Neurosurgery. Freiburg 19–21.

Moriarty, M. J., Mulgrew, S. and Malone, J. R. (1977). Results and analysis of tumour levels of ascorbic acid. *Irish Journal of Medical Science* **146**, 74.

Munson, D., Franco, D., Cubeter, A. *et al.* (1974). Serum levels of immunoglobulins, cell-mediated immunity and phagocytosis in protein-calorie malnutrition. *American Journal of Clinical Nutrition* **27**, 625.

Murray, M. J. and Murray, A. B. (1980). Cachexia: a 'last ditch' mechanism of host defence? *Journal of the Royal College of Physicians of London* **14**, 197.

Pasternak, G. W. (1980). Endogenous opioid systems in brain. *American Journal of Medicine* **68**, 157.

Pert, C. B. and Sugden, S. H. (1973). Opiate receptor: demonstration in nervous tissue. *Science* **179**, 1011.

Pullan, P. T., Clement-Jones, V., Corder, R. *et al.* (1980). Ectopic production of methionine enkephalin and beta-endorphin. *British Medical Journal* **280**, 758.

Reynolds, D. V. (1969). Surgery in the rat during electrical analgesia induced by focal brain stimulation. *Science* **164**, 444.

Rutter, P. C., Murphy, F. and Dudley, H. A. F. (1980). Morphine: controlled trial of different methods of administration for postoperative pain relief. *British Medical Journal* **280**, 12.

Sallan, S. E., Zinberg, N. E. and Frei, E. (1975). Antiemetic effect of delta-9-tetrahydrocannabinol in patients receiving cancer chemotherapy. *New England Journal of Medicine* **293**, 795.

Shaw, D. M. (1973). Biochemical basis of affective disorders. *British Journal of Hospital Medicine* **10**, 609.

Soukop, M. and Calman, K. C. (1978). Vitamin A status and chemotherapeutic responses in cancer patients. *Current Chemotherapy* p. 1296.

Soukop, M. and Calman, K. C. (1979). Nutritional support in patients with malignant disease. *Journal of Human Nutrition* **33**, 179.

Sternbach, A., Janowsky, D. S., Huey, L. Y. and Segal, D. S. (1976). Effects of altering brain serotonin activity on human chronic pain. In *Advances in Pain Research and Therapy*. Ed. by J. Bonica and D. Albe-Fessard. Raven Press, New York.

Subramanian, N. (1977). On the brain ascorbic acid and its importance in metabolism of biogenic amines. *Life Science* **20**, 1479.

Sweet, W. H. (1980). Neuropeptides and monaminergic neurotransmitters: their relation to pain. *Journal of the Royal Society of Medicine* **73**, 498.

Torrey, E. F., Bellenger, J. C., Post, R. M. *et al.* (1979). Headaches after lumbar puncture and insensitivity to pain in psychiatric patients. *New England Journal of Medicine* **301**, 110.

Zaffaroni, A. (1978). *Proceedings of the International Symposium on Science, Invention and Social Change, 19–21 September 1978.* Schenectady, New York.

Zannoni, V. G. and Likans, L. E. (1976). Vitamin C and drug metabolism. *Trends in Biochemical Science* **1**, 126.

The application of symptom control in a teaching hosital

Thelma Bates

A report on the first two years of the terminal care support team at St Thomas' Hospital, London.

The team

During the first two years of its existence, starting in 1978, the St Thomas' Terminal Care Support Team consisted of:
Dr Thelma Bates FRCR
Dr Andrew Hoy MRCP
Mr David Clarke FRCS
Sister Barbara Saunders
Sister Teresa Curtis
Mrs Marylin Thomas (Medical Social Worker)
Rev. Michael Stevens
Miss Bunty Foot (Secretary).

Mode of action

The aim of the Support Team is to improve the care of patients dying from cancer. It does this by advising on the control of symptoms such as chronic pain and by helping to support the patient and his family. The Team does not take over the management of patients and has no beds.

All referrals of patients to the Team are through the patient's consultant or his general practitioner. Domiciliary visiting can usually be accepted if the patient lives within a 6 mile radius of St Thomas' and a medical member of the Team will attend the initial assessment visit if this is requested.

It is the policy that a member of the Team should visit in-patients referred to them every day during their stay in hospital, except at weekends, and regularly at home if required. Sister Saunders works mainly in the hospital and Sister Curtis in the community. Their roles are advisory and they co-operate closely with community and hospital nursing and medical services. Should a patient be discharged, the general practitioner will be contacted and, if he is agreeable, Sister Curtis, who is an experienced district nurse, will visit the patient in hospital prior to discharge and arrange to visit at home. If the patient requires re-admission to hospital, this can usually be arranged promptly through his general practitioner who is always kept fully informed.

The usual number of patients cared for by the Support Team at any one time is 10 in hospital and 40 in the community. An out-patient session is held on Tuesday afternoons in the Radiotherapy Department, at which about 6 patients and their families can be seen. Other patients may be seen in the out-patient department with their referring consultant. The two nurses are the only full-time members of the Team and do the bulk of routine visiting, bringing in other members of the Team as necessary.

There is a weekly meeting of the Team when patients are discussed. The Chaplain and Social Worker attend these meetings and are kept fully informed. They also take part in bereavement counselling, which the Team regards as important. If the patient already has a social worker, the original social worker retains the case. Similarly, if the patient is of another religious denomination, the Chaplain will make sure the appropriate person is informed. The Team has a half-time secretary who maintains prompt communication between the hospital and the general practitioner.

General practitioners and hospital doctors can contact the Support Team at St Thomas' Hospital during normal working hours. At other times one of the sisters will have the Air Call bleep (Tel: 01 828 5621, Code 2791) and one doctor will be available.

Progress

From the annual statistics in Table 5.22 it will be seen that the Support Team is well integrated in the hospital and that during the second year the Home Care Service developed well. At least 80 per cent of patients cared for by the Support Team at any one time are now at home. An increasing number of general practitioners are willing to work within the Team and in 1979 twenty-two of them referred new patients. Good liaison with the district nurses has been established. The number of patients transferred to a hospice has not changed but the Hostel of God, which is the nearest hospice to St Thomas', has been used more often than in the past.

Table 5.22 Statistics

	1st year 1978	2nd year 1979
New patients	207	236
No. of consultants referring patients	29	37
No. of GPs referring patients	5	22
No. of wards involved	26	31
Patients discharged home	93	139
Out-patients seen in the Clinic	269	504
Home visits	301	1339
Patients dying at home	24	46
Patients dying in hospital	105	139
Patients dying in a hospice	22	25
Bereavement visits	7	135
Teaching sessions	59	76
Visitors	44	109

Mrs Thomas, the Support Team's Medical Social Worker, has had considerable experience in bereavement counselling and is currently developing this service. At the moment twenty-five bereaved families are being helped.

Multidisciplinary teaching is considered to be one of the most important aspects of the Support Team's activities. This is achieved indirectly through the Team's mode of action and directly through an increasing number of lectures and tutorials. St Thomas' medical students have not yet been formally included in the teaching programme.

There is both national and international interest in the Team and 109 visitors were received in 1979.

Future development

With the increase in the number of patients cared for at home, a third sister, who will work predominantly in the community, has been approved. She is to be funded by the Special Trustees.

Dr Nell O'Conor was appointed Honorary Registrar to the Support Team for a period of six months which started on February 1st, 1980 prior to taking up the post of Medical Officer at the Hostel of God. She was funded by the Elizabeth Clark Charitable Trust.

6
Hospice Care in Motor Neuron Disease

A review of 100 cases of motor neuron disease in a hospice

Dame Cicely Saunders DBE, T. D. Walsh and Mary Smith

Summary

The notes of 100 patients with motor neuron disease have been reviewed and the experience of the hospice in managing its terminal phases is summarized. The majority of the patients had considerable insight into their condition and welcomed discussion of it. Most patients and families showed an impressive ability to handle their deterioration in a hospice setting. The several benefits of the ready use of small doses of narcotics is described and the use of other drugs, in particular diazepam and the tricyclic antidepressants, is considered. It is hoped that this review may stimulate prospective studies.

Synonyms

Amyotrophic lateral sclerosis; progressive muscular atrophy; progressive bulbar palsy; motor system disease.

Definition

The clinical picture of this disease is of progressive wasting of the muscles, especially those of the upper limbs and those innovated from the medullar, combined with symptoms of corticospinal tract degeneration. In whatever part of the body muscular wasting begins, in most cases it sooner or later becomes generalized. The symptoms of upper and lower motor neuron lesions are usually mixed, although the lower limbs may be spared until the terminal stages. Greenfield (1954) preferred the term amyotrophic lateral sclerosis to motor neuron disease on the grounds that the pathological changes in the spinal cord are not limited to the motor neurons and many American authors use this term as an inclusive one, embracing all varieties of the disease. Motor neuron disease, however, is a better inclusive term (Walton, 1977).

The setting

Our Lady's Hospice in Dublin (1879) and St Joseph's Hospice in London (1905) both included patients with long-term illness in their wards and St Christopher's Hospice (1967) followed this tradition and opened with at least 10 per cent of its ward beds for patients with advanced neurological illnesses. Those with more stable conditions are now rarely admitted as two National Health Service units for the Young Chronic Sick were opened in the vicinity during the 1970s, but the need of patients with motor neuron disease continues and their care has been integrated into the life of the Hospice.

The Hospice opened with six single rooms among 54 beds; all the patients with motor neuron disease were admitted either to nine four-bedded bays or two six-bedded bays and became part of a community which was composed of patients with advanced cancer and a small number of other long-stay patients. Some of them found the constant witnessing of parting and death increasingly hard to bear and were moved into single rooms. Others found the activity of the ward with the continuous traffic and interchange with the nurses greatly outweighed this.

Mrs M. R.'s daughter-in-law wrote an account of Mrs. M. R.'s sixteen-month stay, all of which was spent in a six-bed bay.

'My anxiety was dispelled on my first visit. I can remember vividly, arriving at the Hospice a few hours after Mollie's admission, walking into reception with a child of 15 months in my arms and . . . I was not just told where to go, I was shown . . . where Mollie's bed was, as if she had been there for years . . . the welcome and good impression created by that initial meeting lasted with us until the end.

'There were six beds in Mollie's ward but at no time did Mollie or her visitors feel any lack of privacy. Edward was 15 months when she arrived and Nicholas was born 6 months later . . . Mollie was able to have her home life brought to her, seeing her grandchildren grow up—through breast feeding to potty training and play to reading—and all this happened round her bed . . . Children are a terrific therapy and conversation is never at a loss . . . we were never made to feel embarrassed by having young children in the ward and patients, staff and the children alike used to look forward to the visits.

'Weekend outings were encouraged and the care with which Mollie was made up before we arrived was a tremendous morale booster for her . . . Any day out was encouraged and talked about for some days afterwards which made Mollie feel far less hospitalised.

'Monday at St Christopher's is the only non-visiting day. From our point of view it was a real day of rest. We were able to be at home and not feel guilty that we were not visiting. Being honest, we really appreciated it. But directly Mollie's brother was over from Holland on a Monday he was welcomed as on any other day, given lunch and allowed to stay as long as he wanted. This was typical of how there were rules and no rules.

'Visiting at St Christopher's has left many genuinely happy memories. Being there enabled Mollie to enjoy the last months of her life as much as she could . . . and I missed visiting the Hospice after Mollie died, as it had become part of our life. Edward, who is now three, still insists on our driving past and he loved his visits . . .' (Rusling, 1976).

No patient started in a single room was then moved out to a bay. Some admitted to a bay later moved to a single room when one became available, either permanently or for a break, and weekend outings and holidays have always been encouraged. Patients admitted to the ward of twelve single rooms opened in 1978 have not normally moved to another ward where they would have to become accustomed to a different staff team. In our experience both single and ward beds should be available and many patients balance their individual and community needs better when they have started hospice life in a bay and only then move to a room of their own.

One such patient wrote:

'Loneliness is not so much a matter of being alone as of not belonging. Everyone needs person-to-person contact. To be included in conversations in your presence, a smile, a nod, a wave, any socially acceptable gesture takes little effort and no time. People just drop in for a chat or to give me the latest ward news and, dare I say it, even the occasional moan. Unless they are very good actors I have the feeling that mostly they come because they want to, which is good for my ego.' (Holden, 1980).

It is all too easy to walk past the room of a patient with whom communication is difficult and studies have shown that dying patients tend to wait longer for their bells to be answered than those who are known to be recovering. Once these patients have taken part in the traffic and interchange of a bay they are known to the staff and ways of communication have been developed.

The patient population

Forty men and 60 women are included in this survey. The sex incidence of this disease has an overall majority in favour of the male in the proportion of 3 : 2. This discrepancy is probably due both to the greater capacity of women to care for their disabled spouses or parents and also to the proportion of beds for men and women in the Hospice. Recent alterations now give greater flexibility. Twenty-eight men and 33 women were admitted directly from their homes and 12 men and 27 women were transferred from hospitals. In both cases the diagnosis was made by the neurologists previously caring for these patients (Fig. 6.1).

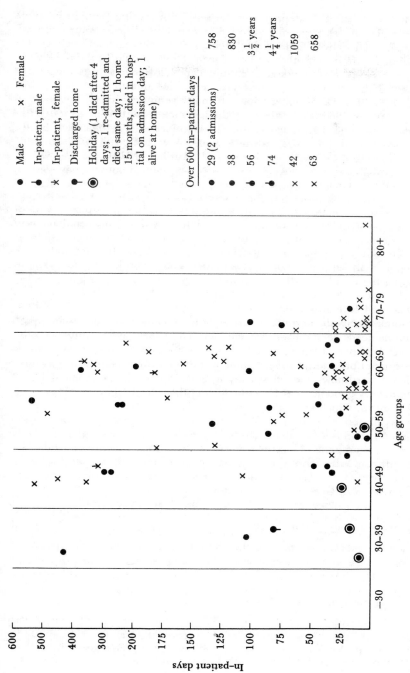

Fig. 6.1 One hundred patients with motor neuron disease (40 male, 60 female).

Motor neuron disease is a disease of late middle life, only occasionally occurring as early as the third decade or as late as the eighth. The median ages in this group were 57 for men (range 29–74) and 64 for women (range 42–91). The median stay was 80 days for men (and ranged from 8 hours to 4½ years (in-patient)) and 32.5 days for women (ranging from 11 hours to 157 weeks).

At present there are eight patients with this disease in the Hospice, two of whom were admitted after the survey figures were finalized. One man with progressive muscular atrophy and no bulbar symptoms has been an in-patient for fifty-three months. Another with a mixed picture has been in for forty-three months after an initial admission of ten days and four months at home before re-admission. One man of 38 years regularly spends two weeks in the Hospice and two weeks at home.

To many readers this may sound like a catalogue of prolonged suffering, but the recent comment of a neurologist visiting the Hospice, 'A most dreadful disease!' was countered immediately by a nursing auxiliary who has worked here for ten years, 'But they are such splendid people.' This is the considered opinion of the Hospice as a whole, for the staff have developed much respect for these patients and confidence and skill in helping them to 'strengthen the things that remain'.

There are few studies on the management of this disease (Norris, 1975; Editorial, 1976a; 1976b; Goodwill, 1976; Rosin, 1976) and most textbooks, in pointing out that symptomatic therapy is all that can be offered, give little space to considerations of such treatment in any detail (Clifford Rose, 1977; Walton, 1977). We emphasize the major difference that a determined programme of symptomatic treatment coupled with a positive attitude can make to a patient's quality of life and to the support of the family, and offer this view as a stimulus to further work in this field.

Length of illness

The rate of progress of this disease shows considerable variation. Of the 100 patients considered in this review, 11 went downhill rapidly and the entire course of the disease was less than one year. Nine men and 14 women had a history of more than three years before they were referred to the Hospice. The remaining 26 men and 34 women had histories of between one and three years before admission. Division into different patterns of disease is somewhat arbitrary, even at the earlier stages of the disease, and nearly all patients presented a mixed picture by the time they were admitted to St Christopher's.

Reasons for admission

These were both medical/nursing and social (see Table 6.1). Paralysis was usually widespread and communication was often difficult; although many of the relatives and friends were frail and/or elderly, most had achieved an impressive level of caring. Nine men and 15 women admitted from home died within one month, having remained at home long after admission would have seemed imperative. In this group only two women had a history of less than one year. Our impression is that because there is no mental impairment this disease is frequently less devastating to families than either multiple sclerosis or cerebral tumour and, although the sheer physical burden made relationships difficult, most showed great resilience and powers of adjustment. The wife of a young man who had managed at home for eight months after an initial admission of three months said when she came back to ask for his re-admission, 'What we have together now is so good that I couldn't bear to lose it if I became worn out and irritable.' Some relatives had continued an almost unbelievable routine of day and night care, often with minimal help from the community services and naturally found it difficult to give up this role. Others shared care gladly

Table 6.1

	Males	Females
Social status		
Relatives/friends to care	33	41
single	2	5
married	27	29
widow(er)	1	7
divorced	3	—
Lived alone	7	13
single	6	5
widow(er)	1	5
divorced	—	3
Communication		
No speech	6	22
Slurred or difficult speech	21	26
Able to speak	13	12

Most who could speak did so slowly and deliberately and eventually had difficulty. One female patient had difficulty because of breathlessness.

Social problems	6
Single (age 91 in OAP home)	1
Married	5
Husband abroad	1
Husband in Scotland	1
Husband violent	2
Not on speaking terms	1
Separated	1

with the ward staff. A nurse wrote of the young couple quoted above, 'His wife visited him regularly and frequently. She would sit close to him, chatting, reading, feeding him and then before leaving she would settle him down comfortably for the night in a deft and capable way which none of the nurses could match; she knew just how he liked to be.' (Church Information Office, 1975).

'All the services of the community became involved with the needs of one Nigerian family. Mrs A. enabled her six-foot husband to remain in his own home for two years after he was virtually quadraplegic. He was determined to remain at home as the strong father to his three young children as long as possible and the Hospice Domiciliary Team were involved with occasional visits. He was admitted for a two-week break 15 months before his death and visited (at his suggestion) one afternoon with his whole family to view slides and discuss a lecture with us a month before his sudden death. At that time his speech was only limited to a slight degree by poor respiration and there was an impressively good relationship with his children who had learned to pick up his signals and give skilful and unobtrusive help. He was still able, with total immobility, to reign from his wheelchair. Four weeks later he collapsed with acute respiratory failure at home on Christmas Day and died in the Casualty Department of the teaching hospital that had continued his follow up ever since the disease had been diagnosed. A decision not to institute Intensive Care Unit type treatment in such an event had been made at case discussions much earlier. The hospital social worker who had helped to co-ordinate the multifaceted support required by this man and his family reports that his wife, who had successfully given him the limelight throughout his illness, had returned to work as a secretary and that the children are all doing well.'

Only 10 men and 10 women were visited at home by the Hospice Domiciliary Team before admission and a further 5 were seen in their previous hospital. Within a few years it had become widely known that the Hospice would welcome these patients and assessment visits were not considered necessary for most patients. Although requests for help came from outside the locality, admission was usually limited to those whose families could visit easily. Not all suitable patients could be admitted as it has been the usual policy to limit the number of these patients in each ward to two except in a crisis.

Management

The problem of telling

'"Do you think you could reorientate your thinking and change your way of life completely?" My reply to the doctor who asked me this question was that I thought I could but only if I knew the extent to which I would have to do this . . . I am very glad that the doctor answered my questions fully and honestly, even to the point of telling me that I would need to be with people who were prepared to do everything for me. Being told that the disease was a progressive one enabled me to do things while I could and not leave them in the hope that I would soon be feeling better.' (Henke, 1968).

'I could not live with a lie . . . I have never regretted telling (my wife) because we have always been able to discuss any problems and work things out together.' (Carus, 1980).

' . . . the dread diagnosis of motor neuron disease. I did not tell my patient . . . I told his wife the diagnosis and she was adamant that her husband must not be told . . .' (This patient travelled widely to receive electrical stimulation and to talk about it . . .) 'he never lost hope. He was sure that he would ultimately win.' (Farn, 1980)

There are many opinions about telling patients of their diagnosis and prognosis and little evidence from studies to sharpen one's intuition as one tries to decide what a particular person wants and needs to know and can handle. A recent paper concerned with patients with terminal cancer cared for in four different settings found that they were least anxious and depressed where communication was frank and where they were given answers to their questions (Hinton, 1979). Terminal cancer has occasional, unexpected regressions or may respond to a final attempt at treatment and any doctor who has worked in a hospice will have a number of such patients to quote if it seems right to add hope and optimism to a poor prognosis. At best, motor neuron disease may have a temporary remission during which time the disease ceases to progress, but this is rare. Many doctors believe that such a prognosis is too bleak to be contemplated in full by anybody and while telling the truth to a responsible relative they give qualified and more optimistic information to the patient. 'In order not to destroy all hope, I believe that it is best to say also that the condition progresses slowly up to a point but then usually becomes arrested, and may even subsequently improve spontaneously, while making it clear that no one can predict when and if arrest will occur. Comparatively few patients seem to be aware of the deception, even to the end.' (Walton, 1977).

Such a policy does not preclude further questioning from the patient and the later giving of a more realistic prognosis by the doctor. We have found that most of our patients have considerable insight into what is happening. Some reveal this to us on admission and others realize later what is happening and may feel ready to discuss it with us.

It is not easy to give figures for the insight of these patients. The truth may be implied but not discussed, may be deliberately avoided or spoken of apparently realistically but with no real comprehension. Above all, insight may change from week to week or from day to day and certainly from person to person. Nevertheless, an attempt has been made from the notes and the writer's memory to give an estimate of varieties of insight in Table 6.2.

We have found there are some aspects of this deteriorating condition that can be discussed helpfully. Patients have been glad to have it re-affirmed that the disease is not multiple sclerosis, which is often known and greatly feared and that it will not affect sight or hearing or mental capacity and that

Table 6.2

Insight	Men	Women
Recorded as total (diagnosis and prognosis)	20	24
Estimated as partial (diagnosis but ? prognosis)	8	16
Obviously knows very little	2	13
Very unrealistic/denial	6	—
Unable to make estimate	4	7

few people are likely to suffer the pain of bedsores or the indignity of incontinence. Above all, we can promise that each problem that arises can be tackled with the confidence born of experience and that we will always be available. We find that this degree of frankness does not deter those who wish to retain hope for a remission, a 'breakthrough' in treatment, or even a 'miracle'.

In our opinion, unwelcome information should never be pressed upon patients, but frustration and desperation are more likely to be caused by too little information than by too much. If the subject does not arise until late in the illness, the patient may then greatly need a serious discussion, however long it may take. Sharing fears can help sort those that are realistic from unrealistic horrors, and the main problems for the patient may well be those that can be dealt with constructively. It is often important that this should be discussed by the doctor and nurse together with the patient.

The capacity of most people to adjust gradually to an unwelcome situation and finally to face it has given the staff courage to trust them with truth when it has been demanded. We have rarely had cause to regret this.

Control and relief of symptoms

The symptoms commonly encountered are listed in Table 6.3, with summarized comments on their relief. Wherever possible, crises such as choking and panic attacks should be anticipated and avoided by imaginative management and sometimes by prolonged discussion. Although the pharmacology is not extensive, some drugs are of well-tried value. Some are used for more than one reason and for different effects. For example, narcotic drugs for dyspnoea, misery, anxiety, insomnia, hunger and thirst as well as for pain: 30 men, 54 women; diazepam for fasciculation, spasticity, cramp and anxiety: 25 men, 38 women; tricyclic antidepressants for depression, sadness, insomnia, with the extra benefit of anticholinergic side-effects: 18 men, 22 women.

The use of narcotics

The confident and skilled use of small doses of narcotics (preferably orally) can transform the management of this disease. (Editorial, 1976b). They

Table 6.3

Symptom	Comment	Therapy
Bowels Constipation (common)	Debilitation, dehydration drugs, immobility, low-roughage diet all contribute. Prevention preferred	Glycerine suppositories, disposable enema, stool softener + peristaltic agent, e.g. Dorbanex, manual removal. Bethanechol
Diarrhoea (unusual)	Rule out constipation with overflow	Codein 30–60 mg prn
Cough	Occasionally a problem, particularly at night, usually unproductive because of loss of muscle power. May be terminal problem—many die with bronchopneumonia	Physiotherapy, positioning, hot drinks—if can tolerate, mouth care. Linctus codein or other narcotic, especially at night. Antibiotics should be considered but not always used, especially late in disease. Suction is counterproductive. Tipping and banging are addictive, possibly prevent pneumonia and gratuitously prolong the terminal phase
Decubitus (uncommon) 8 men; 8 women	Can be extremely painful. Prevention preferred. Nearly all present on admission	Regular position changes, ripple bed, sheepskin. Regular skin care and massage with oil and spirit. The ward-favourite applications and methods

Table 6.3 cont.

Symptom	Comment	Therapy
Dysarthria (common) (see Table 6.1)	Our total concentration required. Trust their persistence and patience—staff get tired before patients stop trying. Talking may first improve and then fail. Find best time of day or punctuate with rest. Help them to communicate somehow	Speech therapy, physiotherapy, writing aids, electric typewriter etc. Possum and similar aids. Individual ideas and tricks. Encourage to talk 'telegraph' style, i.e. short sentences, short conversations. Confirm each word as spoken and never pretend to understand when you don't
Dysphagia and choking (common) 8 men; 33 women Serious swallowing difficulties 13 men; 45 women + choking attacks 8 men; 28 women	Combination of muscle weakness, inco-ordination and spasticity. Variable and fear exacerbates. Idiosyncrasies abound. Semisolids often better than fluids. Confidence most effective therapy. Late admissions present most difficult problems. Little time to establish own routines of prevention. None of present 8 in-patients is choking at present. An unhurried discussion of this problem may greatly alleviate this	Feed slowly with total attention. Learn where to place spoon. Liquidize items individually. Avoid hot or spicy foods. Ice cubes before. Hot plate. Eliminate non-essential drugs. Crush tablets and mix with ice cream. Scrupulous and frequent mouth care. Physiotherapy and speech therapy. Prostigmine/neostigmine 15 mg 2, 3 or 4 times a day + atropine 0.4–0.6 mg more valuable early in disease. For a severe attack, hyoscine 0.4 mg + opiate drug i.m. stat. This may produce some amnesia after the event. Rarely, consider tube feeding, gastrostomy, oesophagostomy. These may prolong life gratuitously. Crycopharyngotomy—not enough evidence yet to assess this

Table 6.3 cont.

Symptom	Comment	Therapy
Dyspnoea (common) 25 men; 35 women	Often associated with anxiety. Progressive with most patients terminally ill. Acute respiratory failure ± pulmonary embolus requires immediate sedation. Do not tip, clap and suck—self-perpetuating/escalating. Do not do tracheostomy. Do not aspirate. Bronchodilators not indicated unless concurrent disease	Calm and assurance. Physiotherapy, windows, fans. Careful individual mouth care. Positioning, speech therapy. Consider antibiotics in early stages, re-consider later, do not give terminally. Use small doses of narcotics freely. Terminally, nearly all need narcotics orally/injection. Diazepam 10 mg for earlier acute attack, narcotic + hyoscine 0.4–0.6 mg for terminal dyspnoea
Hunger and thirst (uncommon where narcotics are being used for other symptoms)	Thirst = symptom (unpleasant). Dehydration = metabolic state (may be asymptomatic). Nasogastric tube, gastrostomy, oesophagostomy are only rarely justified and never in terminal stages. Should be considered for bulbar palsy alone	High-calorie liquids and semisolids. Frequent, small drinks. Scrupulous mouth care. Narcotics control hunger pangs
Insomnia (common)	Often a major problem. Adequate sleep needed. Causes include inability to change position or to fidget, which may lead to pain, e.g. in back and joints, fasciculation and cramp. Unhappiness. Fear of not attracting attention	Attention to physical and mental distress. Routine rituals, warm-water bottle, drinks, micturition. Position changes—frequent and favourite. Hypnotics: nitrazepam, dichlorelphenazone. Tricyclic given at night as sedative. Narcotic analgesics. Indomethacin suppositories at night. Light-touch call buzzer. Foster patients own system. Diazepam for fasciculation. Quinine 300 mg for cramp

Table 6.3 cont.

Symptom	Comment	Therapy
Pain (see Table 6.5)	Arises from lack of movement and poor muscle tone. Spasticity and cramp. Less of a problem than multiple sclerosis	Physiotherapy. Non-steroidal anti-inflammatory drugs. Frequent position changes—own idiosyncrasies. Diversions of all kinds. Analgesics—dextropropoxyphene Co etc. Narcotic analgesics (see below). Muscle relaxants, diazepam, dantrolene sodium, baclofen. But all muscle relaxants tend to increase weakness and there must be search for the critical dose or a compromise. Cryo-probe used once effectively for localized pain
Salivation; secretions } (common)	Distressing—humiliating anticholinergic effects of drugs often welcomed here. Terminal secretions respond if medication given at early stage	Atropine 0.3–0.6 mg bd or prn. Beware rendering sputum too viscid. Watch for eyesight. One patient went blind on atropine 0.6 mg tds temporarily. Hyoscine 0.4–0.6 mg + narcotic prn for terminal secretions. Bisolvon helps a few patients. Patients develop own ways of coping with tissues etc.
Tiredness (common)	Often extreme. Exhaustion may pressage sudden deterioration and death	Prednisone 5 mg tds occasionally used to help appetite and feeling of well-being in earlier stages of disease. Vitamins probably only a placebo effect, but are sometimes welcomed. Watch for and use but do not over-extend activity

Table 6.3 cont.

Symptom	Comment	Therapy
Urinary problems (uncommon) Hesitancy/retention 7 men; 2 women	Catheters may occasionally be used for convenience, e.g. very heavy women	Watch for need for frequent help and for incipient retention. Bethanechol (Myotonin)
Incontinence 7 men; 4 women		
Catheter on admission 2 men; 2 women		
Additional pathology, e.g. menorrhagia	Good general medicine. Consultation with all relevant disciplines as required	

may be used as effective tranquillizers and hypnotics at quite an early stage. The young woman who wrote the article quoted above (Henke, 1968) relaxed by day and slept well on oral diamorphine 2.5 mg tds after finding that more than 2 mg of diazepam and a variety of hypnotics all made her feel doped and heavy. Until forty-eight hours before she died twenty-four months later, she was receiving 5 mg diamorphine tds which both she and the ward staff thought was still effective.

Diamorphine was originally the narcotic of choice in the Hospice, its use based on the unsubstantiated clinical impression formed by the team at St Joseph's Hospice. It was used while awaiting the controlled clinical studies which Twycross was invited to carry out at St Christopher's. He found that, given regularly by mouth at individually optimized doses with a phenothiazine, there was no clinically observable difference between morphine and diamorphine. Morphine was therefore substituted for diamorphine for all oral medication in St Christopher's in May, 1977. The latter drug was kept for injection use because of its greater solubility and therefore potentially smaller volume where larger doses were required. These were not needed for this group of patients and Table 6.4 illustrates the maximum doses of diamorphine given by injection to these patients.

Table 6.4   Maximum (and final) dose of diamorphine

Dose (mg)	Men	Women
2.5	12	19
5	10	21
7.5–10	3	9
15–20	1	5
30	1	—
Total	27	54
Median length of time	11	3
range	1–55 days	1 day–2 years

Three patients received oral morphine and no injections. In all, 84 patients have received narcotics. Three of the present in-patients are on oral morphine at this time.

The pains listed in Table 6.5 were relieved. The 'aches and pains' were often well controlled by the use of physiotherapy and by drugs of the non-steroidal anti-inflammatory group in the earlier stages; narcotics were usually added later for this and other symptoms.

Narcotics were given for distress of various kinds and were used to relieve dyspnoea, misery and frustration, restlessness at night, pain and occasionally feelings of hunger. Some patients received them initially at

Table 6.5   Pain

Men			Women		
Stiffness and aching		7	Aches and pains		14
From bedsores		4	From bedsores		5
Spasms and cramps		4	Cramps and stiffness		5
In limbs		3	Shoulders and back		2
From urinary calculus		1	Colic		2
After micturition		1	After micturition		1
			Sciatic		1
Hunger pangs		1	Hunger and thirst		1
Mental anguish		1	Discomfort from catheter		1
Total		14	Total		31
A few patients had pain in more than one site			One patient had two pains		

night only, with excellent effect. The increase of dose was slow, usually rising in increments of 2.5 mg diamorphine or 5 mg morphine. Cocaine was omitted from the oral mixture in 1977 on the evidence of controlled trials. Alcohol was omitted in 1977 and some patients were glad to take their own drink of choice in the wards and some were regular attenders at the Hospice bar.

Injection diamorphine with chlorpromazine, diazepam and/or hyoscine was used for terminal distress of any kind. Twenty-six men and 50 women had one or more injections. A few patients were very afraid of choking and they knew that an injection of diamorphine and hyoscine was ready at their bedside for immediate help in a crisis. Of the 100 patients, 94 have already died, only 1 in a choking attack.

Opiate drugs are unrivalled in the treatment of terminal motor neuron disease. Used skilfully, orally for preference, they ease distress as no other drug does and the duration of treatment of some of these patients serves to refute the belief that this is a way of shortening life. Control of distress at times appears to lengthen life; certainly it makes it more tolerable. On occasions, however, our commitment to relieve suffering may lead us to take what we consider an acceptable risk.

Death

Table 6.6 gives the modes of death of this group of patients. Confident management and experienced symptom control have enabled nearly all these patients to die peacefully. The most common clinical picture is of a sudden rapid deterioration (i.e. within one week), frequently beginning with an upper respiratory infection and followed by increasing exhaustion and dyspnoea. Distress is relieved by the use of narcotics, combined with

Table 6.6   Mode of death

	Men	Women
Slow	10	18
Quick	24	37
within 24 hours	10	7
In-patient	2	3
Discharged	4	2
a) to home	3	both died at home
alive	2	(1 month later and 1 year later)
died (quickly in hospital)	1	
b) to hospital (died there 9 months later)	1	—

either chlorpromazine or diazepam. Hyoscine is added for any acute crisis or for the relief of excessive salivation and terminal bronchial secretions. Of the 10 post-mortem examinations carried out early in the series, 6 patients had widespread bronchopneumonia. The 4 other *post mortems* carried out among this group revealed the following diagnoses:

    pulmonary embolus
    pontine haemorrhage   )
    coronary artery thrombosis)
    massive haemorrhage from chronic gastric ulcer
    acute respiratory failure.

How these patients died
The following case histories are typical.

    Miss E. H. (see above) was one in whom the common diagnosis of bronchopneumonia was confirmed by post mortem. After many months of slow deterioration during which she had courses of antibiotics for a series of chest infections she developed yet another cold (their usual precursor). The following brief history is taken from the ward daily notes.

10.12. Developing cold with nasal congestion + + , saliva + +
16.12. Nasal congestion at night only now.
17–19.12. Brighter. Up and out in the garden (well wrapped up!)
20.12. Generally weaker. Voice poor with her continuing cold.
22.12. Cold worse. In bed. Asked to see a doctor and told her that this time she did not wish to be given antibiotics.
24.12. Has had good nights, although weaker but now poorly and frightened. Says she can't cope with cough + + O.E. Bronchopneumonia. Diamorphine 2.5 mg given by injection with chlorpromazine 12.5 mg 4-hourly. A quiet night though poor sleep. N.B. This patient had been receiving diamorphine by mouth for 24 months with an increase in dose

from 2.5 mg to 5 mg only. The equivalent was given by injection and was still able to control the distress of breathlessness and unproductive cough. 25.12. Distressed breathing at times. Diamorphine 2.5–5 mg with chlorpromazine 12.5–25 mg given 4-hourly. Barely conscious at 19.00 hours. Diamorphine 10 mg with hyoscine 0.4 mg. 23.05 when became restless. Died peacefully 23.59.

It is essential to control any distress in breathing to the end, including the time when the patient is already unconcious. The medication here should be seen in the context of its use over the previous twenty-four months.

Mrs M. R. (see above) died in a manner typical of the group of sudden deaths. Her illness had progressed inexorably but almost imperceptibly for many months. After a successful outing she was particularly exhausted and she took an unusual day in bed, followed by another afternoon out. The next day increased salivation was noted and then, on sitting out on the commode, she suddenly vomited copiously with considerable distress. After diamorphine 2.5 mg with hyoscine 0.4 mg by injection she rested peacefully but her condition deteriorated rapidly from then on. She continued to dribble saliva and it was found that she required injections of diamorphine 5 mg at 4-hourly intervals to keep her resting quietly. This continued for the next 16 hours but she then became distressed after only 2½ hours and was given a further diamorphine 5 mg with hyoscine 0.4 mg. She was alert enough to be bed bathed but she then became unconscious and died quietly 3½ hours later with her daughter beside her.

Mr G. E. is typical of the 27 patients whose illness ended without either a rapid deterioration or an obvious chest infection.

After a history of about three years and an admission of two weeks Mr G. E. spent more than four months at home, being visited many times by the Hospice Domiciliary Team, working alongside his own doctor and his primary care team. He had recently developed some difficulty in swallowing and had lost nearly all function in both his arms.

After his re-admission on 15.1.76. the summary of his notes reads:

'Settled happily into the ward. Very pleasant and co-operative. Voice soon became weaker; became depressed at times but very undemanding. Turned as necessary, sometimes more frequently than every 2 hours. Found sitting out in a chair very exhausting and tired easily by early February. Manual removals necessary. Looked pale and was rather subdued by the end of February; obviously anxious about his increasing weakness. Bowel problems continued, various aperients tried. Nausea and indigestion troublesome from time to time. Chest pain relieved by Mag Trisilicate. Remained very ill, grey and weak, and condition deteriorated steadily. Speech was incomprehensible by 24/3. Difficulty in passing urine. Muscle spasm became severe and swallowing difficult. Deterioration continued and patient died very peacefully at 02.00 hours on 27.3.76.

The drugs given were as follows:

15/1–21/3	Distalgesic	0	2 tabs 4-hourly.
29/1–21/3	Diamorphine	0	2.5–5 mg nocte

22/3–27/3   Diamorphine   /1   2.5–5–10 mg 4-hourly
31/1–20/3   Stemetil   0   5 mg nocte
23/3–27/3   Largactil   0/1   25/25 mg 4-hourly
13/3–22/3   Redoxon   0   1 g bd
Diazepam nocte and prn 5–10 mg.'

Mood

Moods vary in us all and one could hardly expect this group of people to be free of the common swings of emotion and attitude. Their emotional lability appears to us to be little greater than would be expected of a person of normal affect, afflicted by increasing dependence, often coupled with difficulties in communication and the tendency of those around to treat them as mentally deficient because their speech is awkward or absent. We also note that where they cannot easily smile or look daggers, some alternative has to be found.

Some patients fear that their inability to control tears and laughter foreshadows mental deterioration. Most patients have presented with both lower motor neuron degeneration (progressive bulbar palsy) and upper motor neuron degeneration (pseudo-bulbar palsy). The latter leads to an impairment of voluntary control over emotional reactions. It is common to see an inability to stop laughing or crying but we have only rarely met the more distressing inappropriate responses. 'Impairment of emotional control is a disorder of emotional expression and not due to the underlying mental stage.' (Walton, 1977). It is important at some stage to discuss these reactions, to emphasize that the absence of the 'stiff upper lip' is physical rather than psychological and the fact that 'The main reason for not being able to stop is breathlessness and normal breathing is best regained by the understanding shown by the relative or friend who is present when it happens.' (Henke, 1968).

We need to distinguish sadness and frustration from a true depressive reaction and the comparatively low figure for the use of tricyclic antidepressants reflects this. However, as these drugs are frequently good sedatives and patients may benefit from their anticholinergic side-effects, they may well merit consideration more often in the future. It may also be noted that of 15 patients admitted on these drugs, only 4 of them were considered to be depressed on admission. Fourteen patients who were considered to be depressed were not receiving antidepressants. A total of 18 men and 22 women received them during their stay in the Hospice. One of the present in-patients is receiving them at this time.

Table 6.7 shows the predominant moods reported in the patient notes.

Those classified as 'depressed' and 'sad' had good times and those recorded as 'cheerful and/or composed' had bad times but their swings were not so frequent or marked as those classified as 'variable'. Those recorded as 'anxious' included some recorded thus on admission who improved to 'variable' and others who became frightened with terminal breathlessness which was quickly treated. Every patient was frustrated by

Table 6.7

	Men	Women
Depressed	4	7
Sad	10	9
Variable	11	12
Cheerful/composed	8	21
Anxious/frightened	11	11
Too short a time for assessment	6	11
Pre-senile dementia	1	—

Table 6.8

Symptom	Comment	Therapy
Anxiety	General, from increasing dependence. Especially related to dysphagia, choking, dyspnoea. Control better than relief as may lead to escalating distress and panic	Establish agreed routine with good staff hand-over. Discussion and support, medical/nursing/ social/spiritual. Diversion. Watching successful treatment for others
	Confidence in those around often more effective than any medication	Diazepam 2–5 mg bd tds, 10 mg i.m. or i.v. in acute choking or dyspnoea. Prompt dealing in emergency with injection diamorphine 2.5 mg, hyoscine 0.4 mg, promazine 25–50 mg, chlorpromazine 10–25 mg. *NB* desirability of anticholinergic effects, i.e. reducing saliva
Depression	Distinguish from appropriate sadness, which is a normal reaction and can develop adjustment	Attention to any distress, avoid unnecessary dependence
	Listener rather than medication	Discuss problems in full. Attention to communication, diversion, gossip. Tricyclic antidepressants beginning low doses, preferably single dose nocte, morphine orally

their dependence and a few patients have expressed this aggressively. Art, poetry, wordless sounds, stiffness on being moved and electric wheelchairs can all be used in this way. Treatment is summarized in Table 6.8.

Only 14 patients (8 men and 6 women) have been referred for consultation with the Social Psychiatrist, Dr Parkes, who has spent one or two days a week in the Hospice throughout this time. He has sessions with the staff in each of the four wards and is then consulted about other patients, but his comments are not added to the notes. The inability of some patients to communicate with a new visitor at this stage sometimes makes this his only possible contact. His discussions with some families were recorded and are included in the 14 per cent quoted above. Dying of motor neuron disease is no more a psychiatric problem in itself than is dying of cancer, and even the immense frustrations for both the patient and the family of such inexorable deterioration can be handled by an experienced ward team who use the psychiatrist's time for teaching and back up.

A committed team sometimes needs reminding of the importance of privacy for these patients. Although impotence often develops early and normal sexual relations may no longer be possible, there is often a great need for opportunities for uninhibited expressions of tenderness and intimacy. Time is also needed for the working through of mutual frustrations and the long drawn-out griefs of watching and enduring such illness. The detached listening of the chaplain or the social worker will often contain any tendency to over-involvement in a ward and much time in family casework has sometimes been required. The problems of a few patients and their families have called for many team meetings to face and resolve these problems.

During the month before she died, Miss E. H. dictated a short summary of her search for and discovery of meaning in her illness in discussions with the Hospice Chaplain. His comment 'It must be hard to be the wounded Jew when by nature you would rather be the good Samaritan' helped her to find that being there 'simply to receive' and to link others in a common purpose was a sufficient answer.

A faith in a God as fully identified with the wounded as with the compassionate has been found or found again by a number of these patients. A less articulate discovery of peace and fulfilment has been obvious in others. Help in this sphere should be available to anyone who asks, but never in any way imposed. Even a most determined atheist chose to return to the Hospice for Christmas, manifestly free from any feeling of pressure to conform. In the way they have adjusted to adversity many people, both patients and families, have found the creative possibility of loss.

The Ward Team

Nursing is discussed fully below. We advocate team nursing and the establishment of a routine that encompasses daily needs and encourages readiness to drop in for a chat or a salute with word or gesture to reinforce the feeling of belonging that sustains morale on both sides. Long-stay patients and the staff who care for them tend to become involved deeply with each other and the cost of commitment may be high. Concern about the feelings of these patients when there has been a series of deaths in a ward may reveal the nurses' distress at their own repeated bereavements and in sharing this both may find support. The doctor's responsibility is to understand pressures on the team as a whole, to come in any crisis and to take his part in sharing the burden.

Physio-, speech and occupational therapists have all been used freely and their contributions are discussed. Even now it is not necessarily too late for rehabilitation techniques (Sinaki and Mulder, 1978). Movements that are still possible are carefully encouraged, sometimes with surprising results. Weakness increases if no activity is attempted. Trick movements and other special idiosyncrasies may be discovered and special care given to ways of overcoming the increasing difficulties in breathing and swallowing (Clifford Rose, 1976; Goodwill 1976). These therapists often establish a realistic discussion of this disease. Our Physiotherapy Department has been strengthened as the patient load has increased and each patient is normally treated daily for approximately twenty minutes. Attendance by a speech therapist is on a consulting basis; some patients find great benefit in morale if not in intelligibility and these visits have also helped them to cope better with the difficulties of swallowing and in regaining control after emotional distress.

St Christopher's has a part-time occupational therapist and makes extensive use of volunteers here and elsewhere. The design and organizing of aids of all kinds and help in pursuing a patient's real interests in spite of almost total immobility require imagination. Painting, chess, typing, writing or dictating poetry for a workshop, a listening library and informal discussions have been common interests, but this team has involved many in groups as watchers only and has set up a small electric organ, a wine-making set and collage design and are ready to try anything. A patient writes, 'It will not be much use if the patient is simply asked "What would you like to do?" He/she will have no idea what is possible, available, attainable or reasonable without being too demanding. You can find out what makes people tick through normal relaxed conversation, not by inquisition on an obviously limited time scale. Some will need more prompting than others but I have never met anyone not willing to talk about themselves given an interested audience.' (Holden, 1980).

That this review should end with a comment from a patient serves to emphasize that these people, however much they may lose, can still be very much themselves and a vital support to those around them.

The final summing up comes from a London police sergeant who died after two years in the Hospice and who near the end of that time defined his illness to me as, 'No, not a catastrophic illness—a coming-together illness.'

The caring team in motor neuron disease

Dorothy H. Summers

'I came, I saw, I conquered.' These famous words of Julius Caesar were written on a poster fixed to the wheelchair of a patient with motor neuron disease, dressed as Julius Caesar at a 'Wheelchair Rally'—one of the frivolous occasions held in the summer time at St Christopher's. Here was a man, teacher of Latin and Greek, robbed of his status, his chosen career, his independence and finding himself on the receiving end of care instead of giving it to the boys who came under him. Yet he remained a teacher, albeit an unwilling one, to his wife and those of us who cared for him, for he showed us clearly how through the many little deaths of dying, one can still win the final battle. He came for care and, as in any caring situation, a team approach, using the expertise of the physiotherapist, occupational therapist and speech therapist, as well as the doctor, social worker and chaplain, is the only effective way of meeting the individual and diverse needs of each patient. The nurse who is responsible for the day-to-day needs of the situation is the central member of the team. And who is the team leader? The patient.

The hospice approach has always considered the patient and family together and it interests me that many new units have chosen to care for people with motor neuron disease as their long-stay patients, perhaps because their many needs are more likely to be met in a situation where the staff : patient ratio is high. My personal experience of this group of patients dates back to my days as a volunteer at St Christopher's, when as a ward nurse on alternate weekends I really appreciated the continuing presence of such people as Enid, Valerie, Barry and William, all of whom taught me so much. Coming a little nearer in time, I am particularly indebted to Ted Holden who like them has shared so much of his experience with us all, and to our nursing auxiliaries who have allowed me to learn from them.

The nursing needs of patients will always be individual and changing, depending on the stage of the illness and the neurons and muscles affected. However, the approach and attitudes of the care-givers are fundamental.

Principles of care

Two words sum up what the patient needs—control and communication. There is a tendency amongst experienced nurses to feel that 'they know best', as indeed they do in many nursing situations. Nevertheless, it is essential to be open to what the patient wants and, if we allow him to control his own situation, we create a feeling of security and mutual trust. As the disease progresses, the patient becomes increasingly dependent upon the care-givers and it is important that details of his individual management are passed on to every member of the nursing team. It is helpful, especially, for example, when settling a patient for the night, that a step-by-step procedure is written out so that comfort can be quickly and efficiently achieved. Nurses tend to become anxious and frustrated when they do not immediately succeed, and the patient will often say he is comfortable when this is really not true in order to reassure his nurse—though this is not usually achieved either! Nurses should initiate a 'training programme' for each other during which an experienced nurse passes on her expertise by working with someone less experienced. It is quite alarming for a patient to be faced with two nurses, neither of whom knows his individual needs.

There is a real temptation, especially when verbal communication becomes more difficult, to treat the person who cannot speak clearly as though he is deaf, mentally retarded and speaks a foreign language. Nurses need constantly to remind themselves that people with motor neuron disease are in every way normal, except for their increasing limitations in movement, and the more interesting, variable and stimulating the patient's life can be made, the better its quality will be. It is also important that the patient understands that his condition is a progressive one and that he does not postpone things he wants to do in the hope that he will feel stronger next week. Henke (1968) wrote 'I had business and personal affairs to attend to and friends who lived a long way away I particularly wanted to see, and it was very much a matter of going while I could get in a car and speak clearly enough to make myself understood.' Patients should be helped to live each day at the level of their own full potential, and will enjoy not only listening to the conversation of those around, but will identify with other people and to some extent will live their lives through them.

Patient care plan

Families will be able and want to care for the patient initially, but as the disease progresses professional help may be required. We should enlist their help in establishing a routine of care and many will enjoy still being involved in care giving.

Muscle weakness—positioning and independence

When the upper motor neurons are affected the patient has a spastic paralysis and when the lower motor neurons are affected the muscles will be flaccid. The physiotherapist will make an assessment of the muscles affected and will advise us how to avoid causing discomfort when handling patients, how to prevent deformities, and how to enable patients to achieve maximum independence. The aim of physiotherapy for people with spastic paralysis is to prevent deformity, maintaining the fullest range of movement of all joints by active movement or active assisted movement. Special attention will be given to joints concerned with such activities as feeding, dressing and walking. Passive movements are needed if muscle power is lost and signs of stiffness and deformity are present. Individual joints, especially of the fingers, are moved in all directions, always leaving them in the corrected position.

Light corrective or supportive splints may be of some value, but need to be made for the individual patient. In treating joints which have already become contracted, careful stretching within the limits of pain may be employed, but a wise nurse will leave this to the expertise of the physiotherapist.

Attention to posture is important in the management of patients with flaccid paralysis, especially if trunk muscles are affected. Active, active-assisted and passive movements will maintain whatever power is available, and support for ankles and feet when the patient is in bed and the use of walking aids may be helpful. Respiratory muscles are often neglected and patients should be taught how to achieve full ventilation using the diaphragm and intercostal muscles and to cough effectively. For all patients, relaxation is a useful skill which will enable them to cope with respiratory crises.

When approaching a patient with motor neuron disease whose neck muscles are weak, we should not start a conversation or ask questions until we are directly in front and at the level of the patient's face. Such patients develop tremendously expressive faces, and if we are sensitive and attentive, they will give us a clear indication of how things are for them without expressing it in words. One other effect of weakness of the neck muscles is that the head tends to drop forward, making swallowing and breathing more difficult. The careful choice and arrangement of pillows when the patient is in bed and a chair with a high, adjustable head-rest when the patient is out of bed will counteract this tendency and the head should be positioned slightly backwards from the upright. Few patients can tolerate the use of a foam rubber supportive collar as they find it too restricting, but sometimes a head band around the forehead, fixed to the back of the bed or chair, may be helpful. When lifting the head if it has fallen forward, a hand on the forehead and the other at the nape of the neck is the most comfortable for the patient. Patients will often develop for themselves, or can be taught, 'trick' movements to compensate for non-functioning muscles and the combined expertise of the physiotherapist and the occupational therapist will ensure the timely introduction of gadgets and the Possum machine to help to maintain independence for as long as possible.

Physical care—the role of the nurse

Before embarking on any handling of patients, we need to check that we shall not hurt them with our fingernails, watches, jewellery or badges on the front of our uniforms. We must be sure to assemble all our equipment so that we can give undivided and continuous care and not desert them in the middle of a procedure. It is essential to remember that although movement is limited, sensation is totally intact. The touch of those caring for people with motor neuron disease should be gently effective—that is, sensitive enough not to cause hurt, yet firm enough to create a feeling of security. The energy of the patient is at its peak at the beginning of the day, and it is therefore appropriate to plan nursing care to ensure he will not be too tired to enjoy visitors, diversional activities or whatever other events each day brings and patients will appreciate having some say in this and a flexible routine. It is often thought, quite mistakenly, that these people are emotionally labile, because once they begin to laugh or cry it is extremely difficult for them to stop. This is in fact due to weakness of the muscles of expression and tempting though it may be, it is not kind to tell them too many funny stories whilst we are with them.

Because of patients' physical limitations, some parts of the body need special care.

Eyes
There is a tendency for the eyelids to become sore and for debris to collect in the inner canthus of the lids, especially in the morning. It the patient wakes with 'sticky' eyes, the lids should be swabbed with wool swabs and warm normal saline, working from the inner to the outer aspect. When washing the face, if the nurse uses two fingers under a fold of flannel, she will be able to negotiate the eyes skilfully and should be careful not to get soap in the patient's eyes.

Nose
Patients will find it difficult to blow the nose normally and each nostril must be cleaned with a twist of paper tissue or cotton wool, inserted and turned gently, until it is clean. If there is a lot of mucus in the nostrils they are easier to clean using bicarbonate of soda solution.

Sneezing
This is a very difficult occurrence as there is a tendency to bite the tongue or lip. As sneezing is sometimes promoted when the nose is cleaned, a folded tissue could be placed between the teeth to safeguard this.

Moving patients from sitting to the standing position
The patient's feet, clad in safe slippers or light shoes, should be firmly placed on the floor and 'blocked' from slipping by the nurse's foot placed across in front of the toes. The nurse lifts the patient to the standing position by placing her arms under his armpits, being specially aware that the patient's head and face are neither smothered against her nor raised with the chin tilted upwards over her shoulder. The nurse's hands are placed at the back of the shoulders and it is important to avoid a 'bear hug' grip. A pause to steady the balance is then followed by rotation of the feet and trunk and lowering the patient in the same way that any of us sits down—that is, with the buttocks well back on the seat. It is most uncomfortable if the patient is sat too far forward on the seat and the shoulders are pushed backwards, as the centre of gravity is then lost and the

patient is unbalanced. An awareness of the position of the patient's arms during this manoeuvre is essential. It may be appropriate while the patient is standing for another nurse to wash and thoroughly dry the buttocks and groins and to treat pressure areas with an application appropriate to the condition of the skin. Pressure sores are fortunately not often a feature of motor neuron disease, but their prevention is essential; if they do occur patients may need to remain in bed in the lateral position to avoid pressure on the sacrum, and once this has happened it is extremely difficult to achieve their former stage of mobility.

Clothing

This will be chosen on an individual basis by patients, according to the environment, temperature and their own comfort. Light non-restricting clothing, easily put on and removed, is the usual choice, and the ladies particularly will be interested in their appearance and hair style, and will appreciate the help of the nurse or a beautician with make-up. Some patients tend to perspire and will choose absorbent materials, but one man always wore nylon pyjamas at night which slipped easily and gave him more movement in bed.

Excretion

Micturition is usually normal and presents no problems if an adequate fluid intake is given. Bowels may need some help in regulation and most patients prefer the certainty of action achieved by suppositories or a disposable enema to the uncertain action of aperients. Some patients will be able to achieve a normal bowel action by diet and a regular timing and this must be safeguarded and made possible by the nurses.

Nutrition and feeding

Meal times are social as well as nutritional occasions and should be anticipated with pleasure by patients. Their sense of taste is usually very keen and a variety of flavours should be available. Patients will be well advised to avoid spicy foods and sauces which tend to cause them to catch their breath and choke, but piquant flavours such as cheese, tomatoes and strawberries seem firm favourites. The texture and colour of food are also important and initially patients will be able to enjoy food which is cut into small pieces or finely chopped. Later it may be necessary to liquidize meals and if each food is liquidized separately it is much more palatable and attractive. Patients will often fiercely resist the indignity of being fed and will want to manage for themselves as long as possible, even preferring to bend over their food when arm muscles can no longer lift forks and spoons. They should be given privacy to do this and saved from embarrassment.

Specially designed cutlery with thickened handles, angled spoons, plates with a built-up rim against which food can be held and unspillable beakers will all help people to maintain their independence. Because feeding may take some time, a means of keeping food hot is essential and a plate standing over hot water is useful.

When patients need to be fed, the undivided attention of the helper is vital. Distractions at meal times are a great trial to patients and every effort should be made to avoid these. The nurse must concentrate on the task in hand and not gaze out of the window or converse with the patient in the next bed. Choking is one of the patient's greatest fears, and should this happen he should be helped to sit forward and reassured until the coughing attack has passed. The speech therapist will teach patients to control their breathing, particularly when taking a drink and many will prefer to take fluids in a long drink rather than in sips.

Salivation

Excessive salivation resulting in dribbling often occurs and this is well controlled by giving atropine 0.6 mg twice a day. At night time a small absorbent pad placed under the corner of the mouth will keep patients dry and comfortable.

Communication

Of all the challenges presented to the caring team, communication is perhaps the greatest and highlights the importance of establishing a nursing care plan early on while the patient can still tell us what he likes without too much difficulty. Mention has already been made of the importance of being in front and at the level of the patient's face before starting any exchange of information, and one soon gets accustomed to making statements and asking questions in such a way that only a 'Yes' or 'No' answer is required. For example, when discussing the menu—'There is jelly and ice cream or egg custard—would you like jelly and ice cream?'

The speech therapist will be invaluable to both the staff and patients and her advice should be sought to overcome problems of communication. Patients should be allowed time to speak and should be watched attentively as they do so. Short sentences and short regular conversations are more profitable: important information should be exchanged earlier in the day when patients are less tired. The use of ice may help to stimulate muscle movement, and patients may like to suck a small ice cube or to lick an ice cube with the tip of the tongue, while a nurse holds it just beyond the lips. Facial muscles may be stimulated by passing an ice cube from the corner of the mouth towards the ear and then drying the skin. It may also be helpful to wipe an ice cube round the lips and then dry them. These measures do not always help speech but are well worth assessing on an individual basis.

Other ways in which individuals can be helped to communicate are by teaching them to use the Possum machine to work a typewriter and one patient who had some movement in her eyelids was able to blink messages in Morse code.

It must be made possible for patients to summon help when required, and devices to ring an ultrasensitive buzzer which can be operated by whichever muscles still produce some movement can be designed by the maintenance staff with the advice and guidance of the physiotherapist and the occupational therapist.

Diversion, recreation and mobility

Despite the needs of patients for nursing care which will bring them helpers at regular times during the day, there are still many hours when they will be alone. The visits of family and friends will be highlights of the day and other activities can be enjoyed in the company of other patients and the staff. These need not be restricted to the confines of the ward, and the provision of an electric wheelchair will give patients mobility and independence. Outings to theatres and concerts can be arranged, and many places of entertainment make special provision for people in wheelchairs. Car rides, visits home for a day or weekend and even a holiday can be made possible in the earlier stages of the illness and will provide pleasure in anticipation and a welcome change of environment. Music, television and games such as chess are also enjoyed and help to pass long hours of inactivity. Attendance at chapel services and visits from the chaplain will provide for the patient's spiritual needs.

Needs of the family

Our work on the patient's behalf would be incomplete if we failed to include his family under the umbrella of the caring team. To watch a loved one with a progressive condition slowly losing independence and becoming physically more frail is a devastating experience and at times the feeling of helplessness becomes almost intolerable. Families may sometimes feel resentful of the help which professional staff can provide and it is important to enlist their help with patient care when appropriate. They should be encouraged to come and share their feelings when they visit and, although we can do little to change the situation, an understanding listener can be very supportive. It is equally important that we do not intrude on the privacy and intimacy of a family visit as people still need to have time alone together.

Conclusion

Despite their physical limitations, people with motor neuron disease always seem to have an indomitable spirit and give so much to those privileged to care for them. Their needs challenge the expertise of everyone in the caring team to refute the saying 'What cannot be cured must be endured' and to make the enduring a positive and worthwhile experience for everyone.

References

Carus, R. (1980). Motor neurone disease: a demeaning illness. *British Medical Journal* **1**, 455.

Church Information Office (1975). *On Dying Well*. An Anglican Contribution to the Debate on Euthanasia. Church Information Office, London.

Clifford Rose, F. (1976). Motor neurone disease. *Transactions of Medical Society London* 92.

Clifford Rose, F. (1977). *Motor Neurone Disease*. Pitman Medical, Tunbridge Wells.

Editorial (1976a). Management of motor neurone disease. *British Medical Journal* **1**, 1422.

Editorial (1976b). Symptomatic care in motor neurone disease. *British Medical Journal* **2**, 605.

Farn, K. T. (1980). Motor neurone disease. *British Medical Journal* **1**, 791.

Goodwill, J. (1976). Management of motor neurone disease. *British Medical Journal* **2**, 42.

Greenfield, J. G. (1954). *The Spinocerebellar Degenerations*. Oxford University Press, London and New York.

Henke, E. (1968). Motor neurone disease—a patient's view. *British Medical Journal* **2**, 765.

Hinton, J. (1979). Comparison of places and policies for terminal care. Occasional Survey. *Lancet* **i**, 29.

Holden, E. (1980). *Nursing Times* **76**, 1035.

Norris, F. H. Jr. (1975). Recent advances in motor neurone disease. In *Recent Advances in Myology*, p. 522–36. Ed. by W. G. Bradley *et al*. Excerpta Medica, Amsterdam.

Rosin, A. J. (1976). The problems of motor neurone disease. *Age and Ageing* **5**, 37.

Rusling, T. (1976). *St Christopher's Hospice Annual Reports*.

Sinaki, M. and Mulder, D. W. (1978). Rehabilitation techniques for patients with amyotrophic lateral sclerosis. *Mayo Clinic Proceedings* **53**, 173.

Walton, J. N. (1977). *Brain's Diseases of the Nervous System*. Oxford University Press, London and New York.

7
The Hospice Movement Worldwide

Africa

Judith van Heerden

Hospice care in Southern Africa

The third world countries are still struggling to establish primary medical care services in the form of 'barefoot doctors'. Their social structure and extended family systems obviate the anxiety, tension and isolation of the nuclear family of the West, so that it is doubtful whether the need for such a sophisticated system as a hospice exists at this time for the great majority of African nations.

I shall therefore summarize the present hospice situation in the big centres of South Africa and Zimbabwe.

Terminal care groups have been established in the main cities—Johannesburg, Pretoria, Cape Town, Port Elizabeth and Salisbury (Zimbabwe). The distances separating these centres vary between 500, 750 and 900 miles and lack of communication between them contributes to diversity of approach.

Zimbabwe

Salisbury

A resident of Salisbury, Mrs Butterfield, had her interest aroused in terminal care while nursing her own daughter with cancer in 1977. Two years later when in London she made contact with St Christopher's Hospice. Soon after her return to Africa she was able to attend a lecture on 'Death and Bereavement' in Johannesburg at which Dr Cicely Saunders was the guest speaker.

On her return to Salisbury, inspired by this experience, and with the help of university staff, she arranged an exploratory symposium. The public response to this exceeded all expectations. This resulted in the establishment of an organization called 'Island', taking its name from the Devotions of John Donne—'No man is an island . . . every man's death diminishes me because I am involved in mankind'. Their objectives are to work towards establishing a hospice and to conduct an educational programme for professionals, lay workers and the public at large. The Little Company of Mary, whose order was established to take care of the dying, have co-operated in putting at their disposal two four-bedded wards and a single ward in St Anne's Hospital, Salisbury.

South Africa

Pretoria
At present, care of the dying patient seems to be the responsibility of the hospital chaplain, though as far back as 1971 the people of Pretoria saw the need for and initiated research into the feasibility of a terminal care centre. Their objective is a brick-and-mortar hospice. At present they have ground available and plans have been submitted to the authorities for approval and financial backing. They also have the assurance that the National Cancer Association will subsidize on a daily basis those patients who cannot afford the full hospice fees.

Johannesburg
After two false starts, the Hospice Association of the Witwatersrand was eventually established in Johannesburg in mid-1979. A group of highly skilled people, they are motivated, enthusiastic and determined to succeed. In a business-like fashion they started by drawing up a constitution, a mailing list, a newsletter and appointing a glittering array of presidents. They have also been fortunate in obtaining the financial support of some mining houses. More recently they have concentrated on patient care. A part-time doctor and two home-care sisters have been made available by the National Cancer Association, while beds for patients who require hospitalization are provided by a local nursing home. They also have the option to take over the building were it to become obsolete. On average they can at present cope with ten home-based patients.

Cape Town
Patient support is provided by the Hospice Chaplain, Dr Hendrik Venter, and his team at Tygerberg Hospital. Dr Venter did two years postgraduate training in pastoral care overseas, of which he spent two months at St Christopher's Hospice. Ideally, this team aims to be present when the patients are informed that they have cancer, and also when the patient is told that active treatment is no longer indicated. They have also introduced a 24-hour on-call roster for emergency cases. Whenever a serious accident case is expected in casualty, they are informed so that they are present when the patient arrives. Even if the patient is unconscious they are able to give support to the distressed relatives. One wonders why all the large hospitals do not introduce this system.

Port Elizabeth

In 1976 Dr Tom West of St Christopher's visited Port Elizabeth. As a direct result of this visit two wards were set aside for nursing cancer patients, including those requiring terminal care. In these wards open visiting hours were allowed, but more important was the introduction of a four-hourly pain control schedule. Despite these improvements, a group of members of the radiotherapy department was concerned about the lack of emotional support of the patients. It was a visit from St John's Ambulance nurse, Sister Lesley Lawson, to ask for help with patients she was treating on district, that prompted us to more positive action.

Together with Life Line (Samaritans) we ran a pilot project for training counsellors which was attended by doctors, nurses, social workers and members of the clergy. On one occasion we were privileged to have Miss Willans, Matron of St Christopher's, address our group. When Dr Saunders visited South Africa in March 1979, a contingent of six from our group flew to Cape Town to attend the symposium 'Death and Euthanasia' organized by the students of Cape Town University.

From this group was evolved the nucleus of the home-care team whose objective is to provide domiciliary care on a voluntary basis. Sister Lawson has been appointed by the National Cancer Association for home nursing. We refer patients from the radiotherapy department to her and also provide their medication, so that she forms the link between the home and the hospital. We are in daily contact with her and once a week she reports back to a meeting of the team. This arrangement works well and since its introduction the wards have not been as overcrowded. On average, Sister Lawson looks after fifteen patients monthly.

To get our project on a firm footing and for the sake of uniformity and easier communication we have, with minor alteration, adopted the constitution of the Johannesburg group.

What of the future?

We have first to establish the needs of the tribal and of the urban African and to consider the effects of the language and cultural barriers which exist between Black and White, and Black and Black.

South African society is of considerable racial and cultural diversity. Our population comprises several major groups in which there is a wide range of customs and beliefs, lifestyles, educational levels and degrees of sophistication, wider perhaps than any of the industrialized nations of the West. The diversity is compounded by the difference which exists within the major groupings. In the white group (16.5 per cent of the population) the ratio of Afrikaans speakers to English speakers is approximately 3 : 2. The Black people of South Africa can be divided as shown in Table 7.1.

Industrialization has brought in its wake the nuclear family, out of which has developed our modern need for hospice care. Among the rural African there exists an extended family pattern in the form of a kraal consisting of several huts in which live units of the family structure. At the head is the

Table 7.1

	Numbers (thousands)	Percentage
Zulu	6200	31.5
Xhosa	5800	29.0
N Sotho	2000	10.0
S Sotho	2000	10.1
Twana	1600	8.0
Tsonga	700	3.4
Swazi	600	3.0
Ndabele	500	2.5
Venda	500	2.5

father with each of his wives forming a unit. What better means exists for providing financial and social support for the bereaved?

The urbanized African is in a very different position. In the townships are second and third generation Blacks who have become westernized. They are joined by the man from the country who has come to earn a better wage in the city, leaving his wife and children behind. He may take unto himself a 'comforter' and her main function is to prove his male virility. If she does not fall pregnant she is discarded as an insult to him. If she becomes pregnant she is discarded after the birth as a financial burden. Sadly a group of people is created who have no roots and do not belong.

We can help them but there are pitfalls. Our biggest stumbling block is the language barrier. It is difficult enough to establish channels of communication with a common background and tongue. The majority of white doctors are completely dependent on their interpreters. The trained staff who interpret are often more sophisticated than the patients with whom they deal. Technical terms are translated as words but conjure up a totally different word picture. Imagine the country woman in a city hospital. Someone has explained to her the need for an operation and that she will be put to sleep. She has even signed consent for operation. When by 10 o'clock the next morning she is the only one in the ward who has had nothing to eat or to drink, she is outraged. Her dissatisfaction is made clear in a loud voice and chaos reigns in the ward. The technically skilled African sister often does not approve of all 'these goings on'. Even if she realizes what it is all about she is unsympathetic towards 'those people and their ways'. In many cases she has been well taught by the missionary about the evils of superstition. Understanding would tar her with the same brush of ignorance.

In the out-patient department we are still able to distinguish between the rural and the urban African by their dress. Once they have been admitted to the wards and issued with standard hospital bedclothes it is more difficult to know at what level to converse with the patient. Only a small percentage of affluent Africans attend private nursing homes. The majority make use of State-supported hospitals where they are charged a nominal fee and if unable to pay are treated free of charge. The fee includes an examination, investigations, drugs and referral to a specialist if indicated. If the local hospital does not have the facilities to investigate and treat a particular case, the patient is transferred, at the cost of the State, to an institution where such facilities exist.

In the same way patients arrive from outlying areas for radiotherapy. When patients become terminal we try to return them to their home-town before death occurs. The State will transfer patients free of charge, but bodies are the responsibility of the family and transporting the corpse back to where the funeral will be held is exorbitantly expensive for people with a small income. At this stage in South Africa centralized terminal care is, I believe, neither practicable nor desirable.

USA

Janet Lunceford

Hospice in America

Americans have recently been undergoing certain changes of attitude towards death and dying. The need to humanize our health care system, so that room can be made for the growing hospice movement in the United States, is beginning to be recognized. Although the hospice concept is still very new and just starting to evolve in our country, with 'hospice' yet to become a household word, it is evident that interest and enthusiasm are growing throughout the USA. The emergence of an American hospice movement, modelled after St Christopher's Hospice, has undoubtedly stimulated an interest within the US Federal Government in the improvement of care for terminally ill patients and their families, particularly in the area of pain control. The new focus on the psychological and social aspects of terminal illness which has recently become emphasized in our federally funded programmes can also be attributed to the English model of hospice care. The visits and consultations of Dr Saunders and her associates, as well as other English hospice staff, have been instrumental in the development of the hospice movement in the USA. If it were not for Dr Saunders' efforts and the excellence of St Christopher's Hospice, the United States hospice movement would not be where it is today.

The hospice concept has begun a revolution in our American health care system and in the way American people regard terminal illness and care of the dying. Because of the emphasis the hospice approach places on pain control and humane care of the patient and family experiencing terminal illness, even studies and programmes to improve long-term care of chronically ill and elderly patients have come to the forefront of national attention. It is an exciting time for health professionals involved in all areas of health care.

The role of hospice has not yet been determined by the Federal Government, which is still in the process of learning where and how hospice should fit into our system of health care. When it became apparent to the US Congress that their constituents were actively involved in the hospice movement and were seeking support from Congress, the Federal Government stepped in to examine the situation. Consequently, the Department of Health and Human Services (formerly the Department of Health, Education and Welfare) made an initial commitment to explore the hospice concept in the USA. The former Secretary of this Department, Joseph Califano, visited our first established American hospice in New Haven, Connecticut, and it was largely because of his interest and enthusiasm that a number of demonstration projects in hospice were funded.

There is continued interest in the development of hospice at the Federal level. A Hospice Work Group consisting of members of this Department and their agencies involved in some aspect of hospice research or demonstration has been meeting on a regular basis since 1978. A significant development which came out of this widespread grassroots interest was the creation of an Interagency Committee on New Therapies for Pain and Discomfort within the Department of Health and Human Services. In May 1979, the Committee submitted to the President of the United States a report which included an entire section on identified areas of the clinical management of terminal care. We regard the fact that this report gained the ear of the White House as an important step towards furthering the American hospice movement.

In addition to the Interagency Committee on New Therapies for Pain and Discomfort, seven organizations within the Department of Health and Human Services have been active in hospice. Chief among them is the National Institutes of Health, commonly referred to as NIH. From modest beginnings in a one-room Laboratory of Hygiene in 1887, the National Institutes of Health has evolved into one of the world's foremost and most prestigious biomedical research centres, the focal point for Federal biomedical research. Its mission is to improve the health of all Americans. To achieve this goal the NIH conducts biomedical research in its own laboratories; provides grants to non-profit organizations and institutes for research and for medical education, including improvement or construction of library facilities, buildings, equipment and other resources; and provides grants for the training of research investigators and supports biomedical communications through programmes and activities of the National Library of Medicine.

The National Cancer Institute (NCI) is one of eleven institutes within the NIH, and is the first Federal Governmental agency to engage in the support of a hospice programme. In 1974, the NCI awarded a three-year contract to Hospice, Inc., now known as the Connecticut Hospice, in New Haven, Connecticut. Of all of the existing programmes, the Connecticut

Hospice has probably come closest to the ideal set by St Christopher's. Dr Sylvia Lack, Medical Director of the Connecticut Hospice, has contributed enormously to the hospice movement across the country through her dedication and leadership.

The success and worth of the Connecticut Hospice programme stimulated the NCI's interest in further exploring the hospice concept, and three hospice programmes were funded—the Kaiser-Permanente Hospice in California, the Riverside Hospice in New Jersey, and the Hillhaven Hospice in Arizona. Each developed a comprehensive home care programme with a back-up in-patient facility.

The Kaiser-Permanente Hospice is located in the Southern California region of the United States. It is a large, prepaid, group practice medical care delivery system known as the Health Maintenance Organization. The programme serves approximately one million people in the Los Angeles area, which constitutes about 12 per cent of the total population. As an extension of the programme's commitment to provide a total range of care for its members, a hospice programme emphasizing home care was opened in June of 1978. Patients are referred to the hospice programme by physicians working in four major medical centres in the area. The medical management of patients referred to this programme is assumed by the hospice Medical Director and the hospice physician.

The Hillhaven Hospice is located in Tucson, Arizona, serving a population of approximately 500 000 people in a retirement community setting. It is a fully comprehensive programme which began operation in April 1977. Hillhaven Hospice was the first hospice venture by a major proprietary nursing home chain, Hillhaven Inc. of Tacoma, Washington. In 1981, the hospice was moved to a Tucson hospital, St Mary's, and is now designated St Mary's Hospice.

Riverside Hospice is located in Boonton, New Jersey. The hospice programme began operation in January 1977, and serves approximately 402 000 of the people in the northern part of the State. Riverside, formerly free-standing, is now located in Riverside Hospital, a small community hospital. Community physicians refer patients to these programmes and for the most part remain the patients' primary care physicians, with the hospice Medical Director and physician serving as consultants and as a resource for symptom control.

The National Institute of Aging, another part of NIH, is also studying hospice and is currently funding studies in the area of 'aging and bereavement'. The study of bereavement in this country is a fairly recent focus of study by the Federal Government.

Other Federal agencies studying hospice include the Administration on Aging, which has funded three hospices; the National Center for Health Statistics Research, which is conducting a study on hospice home care; the Health Resources Administration, which is supporting two hospice educational programmes, including an interdisciplinary team training programme and a hospice training programme for nurses; the National Institute of Mental Health, which has awarded three training grants in relation to hospice, including funds to produce a film about hospice, and demonstration training projects for hospice staff and volunteers; and the Health Care Financing Administration studies on reimbursement for hospice care.

Before describing the Health Care Financing Administration (HCFA) hospice study, I would like to explain a little about our health care reimbursement system. For some years now the Federal Government has set aside public funds to provide care for persons who do not have private health insurance or the means to pay the extremely high cost of medical care in the USA, and for persons aged 65 years and older who are at this same disadvantage. These public funds are offered through programmes known as Medicaid and Medicare. Without Medicaid and Medicare reimbursement, hospice staff would not be fully paid for their services and consequently the hospice programmes would not remain solvent for long.

Unfortunately, the current policies of Medicare and Medicaid insurance prohibit full reimbursement for hospice services such as the administration of drugs for the control of pain or other symptoms in the home, or bereavement visits by hospice staff. In the interest of responding to the public's complaints about this lack of reimbursement for hospice care, twenty-six operational hospices were selected by the Health Care Financing Administration to participate in a two-year National Hospice Study which allows coverage and reimbursement for all hospice services to Medicare and Medicaid patients. The objectives of this study conducted by Brown University are to determine:

(i) the relative cost effectiveness of care provided in hospice and non-hospice settings;

(ii) the impact of hospice care on the health, well-being and quality of life of terminally ill patients (with advanced cancer) and their families;

(iii) the impact on hospice of Medicare/Medicaid funding; and

(iv) the likely national costs and utilization implications of reimbursing hospice services through Medicare/Medicaid.

The results of this study (to be submitted to the Health Care Financing Administration in the Autumn of 1983) will be critical in assisting the Department of Health and Human Services in making new policy decisions regarding coverage of hospice services under the Medicare and Medicaid programmes. The outcome of this study obviously has the potential for a significant impact on the future of hospice development.

The reimbursement problem is not the only difficulty which hospice leaders must tackle. Starting a hospice in-patient facility is not easy in the USA because it involves more than converting a building or home into a hospice in-patient facility. Federal, state and local regulations and policies must be complied with, and this requires a very lengthy process of applying for a Certificate of Need for a total hospice programme, which means the hospice staff becoming involved in public hearings, testimonials, and a good deal of red tape. Six months is not considered an unusual length of time for obtaining a Certificate of Need and it can take considerably longer. Once the Certificate of Need is granted, applications for licensure must be filed with the state and/or county before a hospice can become an operative facility. Legislative and insurance problems must be tackled as well. Since each state has autonomy within its own separate government, laws and ruling officials, every new hospice must comply with its own state regulations and standards.

A dramatic and fairly typical example of what a comprehensive hospice programme must do to get a home care programme and a back-up in-patient facility operational can be seen in the case of one of the National Cancer Institute's programmes. Hillhaven Hospice (now St Mary's Hospice) in Tucson, Arizona, worked for two and a half years to change the State regulations governing hospital and other health care facilities. They were finally successful in persuading the State to create a special designation which would qualify the hospice as a 'special hospital/hospice' rather than a skilled nursing facility, as it had been originally classified. This creation of a new designation was necessary in order that hospice patients could be admitted directly into the in-patient facility from home, without having to sojourn in a hospital for three days first, as is currently required by law throughout the US in order to receive Medicare reimbursement. Without this special designation, those hospice patients who were dependent on Medicare insurance were subjected to a discontinuity of care by means of a forced admission to a hospital for three days.

Probably the major obstacle in the development of hospice in America is the difficulty in obtaining funds to develop or support initial programmes. Individual hospices seek funds from private sources, voluntary contributions, or as grants from private foundations. However, funding sources are not usually initiators of hospices; it is more normal for individual hospices to be organized first and then to approach the funding organizations to develop their programmes. Funding agencies usually prefer to give money to programmes that have shown potential for growth or demonstrated a high degree of credibility. Because hospice is so new and the Federal Government has still not determined its role in hospice care, funds or low-interest loans for construction or renovation for hospice usage and expansion are rarely available. Each hospice must develop independently. The National Hospice Organization (NHO) is the one unifying organization which offers guidelines and advice on the integral steps to be taken in developing a hospice home care programme and obtaining hospice beds.

The National Hospice Organization is the first private group to provide national initiatives, confront emerging problems and seek appropriate directions for future progress in organizing a national hospice movement. The NHO, which now estimates that there are over 700 hospices operating in the United States, was formed in February 1977. It has already achieved notable successes in developing guidelines in the areas of standards and criteria, education and training, evaluation and research, liaison with other health organizations, public relations and reimbursement and licensure. It has produced an educational film on hospice to be available to the public and for commercial television, and a regularly distributed newsletter to its members on what is happening in the hospice movement across the nation, including the progress of individual hospice organizations, issues in hospice development and administration and current legislative matters. The NHO has succeeded in opening up communications with governmental organizations, the Congress of the United States, the media, the membership of NHO, other national health organizations and the general public—important because many physicians and in particular the oncological medical community are not yet convinced that hospice is a viable alternative form of care for terminally ill patients. To them, hospice is revolutionary and therefore suspect. Some oncologists fear that hospice will deny or interfere with the patient's right to optimal treatment and the most up-to-date methods, while others fear it is a one-way street, possibly leading to an unnecessarily premature death. Often it is the case that such scepticism is diminished once the hospice philosophy and methods are explained, but it may take some years of effort before hospice is accepted by the traditionally oriented medical community.

USA: the next decade

Sister Zita Marie Cotter

Hospice as a human rights movement

Among the most significant contributions of the recent resurgence of the hospice concept of service is its tendency to free persons to become more involved in, and to assume more responsibility for, the circumstances which surround their own deaths and the last illness and death of those they love. The attention and support now accorded them by medical and other health professionals, religious ministers, family and friends, and volunteer helpers, allows those who face serious and progressive illness to experience a more meaningful participation in decisions which affect them in depth at this time. From this viewpoint, the hospice movement may be seen as being well in the forefront of a significant deepening of respect for human rights, and the next decade should hold opportunities for the expansion and diversification of this deeply human role.

It is not unusual now to see notices or pamphlets posted in hospitals, hospices, clinics, nursing homes, rehabilitation centres and other facilities offering care to the sick or disabled, which announcements describe in detail the patients' *bill of rights*. Among these are listed the right to receive safe, considerate and respectful care; to be fully informed by one's physician, if one wishes, of one's diagnosis, treatment and prognosis, in so far as these can be determined; to be sufficiently enlightened as to be able to give an informed consent, or to decline consent, relative to examinations, treatments and medications; to be sufficiently informed as to make an appropriate decision for or against one's own participation in research studies involving experimental drugs or diagnostic procedures; and to have one's request for spiritual support and consolation responded to according to one's wishes.

The hospice movement seems to be an active agent for radical change in the area of simply enabling the realities of death and dying to become acceptable topics of conversation, not only among professional health care groups, but among clergy, psychologists, philosophers, students of every persuasion, co-workers in patient care, patients and their families, and even among chance acquaintances waiting in queues in airports, bus-stations and supermarkets. Not infrequently the focus of such conversations centres on the need to be safeguarded from the scientific and technological possibilities of having one's own dying extended far beyond the time involved in the *natural* process of dying from terminal illness; and, in more recent years, the spectre of the possibility that future expanding government controls, and/or supreme court decisions, may infringe, by way of legalized euthanasia, on one's inalienable right to life. In both instances, the growth and acceptance of the hospice philosophy is seen as a haven offering protection against an invasion of one's innate human rights.

Although by June, 1979 ten states had passed so-called 'death with dignity' legislation, this movement has not grown extensively. A more personal approach, which has many advocates, involves a signed statement, placed in the hands of a trusted family member, pastor or other friend, expressing the request 'that, if possible, I be consulted concerning the medical procedures which might be used to prolong my life as death approaches. If I can no longer take part in decisions concerning my own future, and there is no reasonable expectation of my recovery from physical and mental disability, I request that no extraordinary means be used to prolong my life.' Such a statement, although not considered a legal document, gives a person reasonable assurance of respect for his wishes, within the framework of a shared friendship and value-system.

Taking time in advance to reflect on one's own death and burial seems to be another positive fruit of the openness concerning death and dying engendered by the hospice movement. Such an approach is evidenced in available questionnaire-type folders which allow for personal statements describing one's preference concerning memorial services and funeral liturgies; indicating the desired celebrant, homilist and other participants; the place and type of burial, whether simple or elaborate; permissions for organ donations for transplants, and related information. Space is also provided for information helpful to survivors: the location of personal papers relative to finances, military discharge, pension and insurance benefits, and designation of the executor of one's will. A copy of this folder, completed and dated, can be entrusted to one's pastor or other friend or family member, with a better-than-ordinary assurance that it will be respected. Completion of such a plan at a time when one is well and able, and has time to consider it thoughtfully, relieves a person of this burden at a time of illness, with its associated stresses. This allows a certain relief that these matters can be dismissed in favour of reflection, family sharing, reunion and prayer. A more subtle benefit of this process is the opportunity it offers to look at one's death in real terms and to claim it as one's own, after the manner of a human person, gifted with the capabilities of knowing, loving and choosing a liberating experience befitting one's humanity. As Dag Hammarskjold wrote: 'In the last analysis, it is our conception of death which decides our answers to all the questions that life puts to us. That is why it requires its proper place and time if need be, with right of precedence. Hence, too, the necessity of preparing for it.'

A related human-rights interest which is gaining momentum in the United States and Canada is the movement to inform the consumer about alternatives to the traditional high-cost funeral. Termed 'Memorial and Funeral Society', the association advocates a return to simplicity and economy in funeral arrangements to emphasize the spiritual values of life and death rather than exalting the physical. This movement is being met with widespread response at the level of the local neighbourhood and community, where information and insights are shared in small group meetings.

Recent stirrings give evidence of a movement to reclaim relatives and friends from the spectator role to the more integral services which have long been turned over to professional functionaries. In the remote rural villages of Northern New Mexico, the Spanish-American people have never relinquished the role of family and friends in caring for the dying and in honouring and burying the dead. Here the age-old Penitente brotherhood, rooted in the faith and family bonds which are their heritage from the early Spanish conquistadores, preside at the wake and rosary with traditional Spanish prayer and song, assist the mission priest with reverence at the requiem Mass and, when the coffin has been lowered and the eulogy given by one of the brothers, pick up their shovels and return their brother or sister to the good earth which has been cherished as their mother and nurturer through centuries.

In the Jemez Mountains northwest of Santa Fe is Los Alamos, New Mexico, home of the nuclear research which developed the first atomic bomb, in whose laboratories medical research has pushed back frontiers of healing. Here in a community of eminent scientific education and sophistication, state-wide leadership has been given to a movement to reclaim the freedom to make decisions in favour of simple and inexpensive mortuary and burial services, and to retain the direction of these arrangements. In both these instances, a neighbourly love and concern supports the bereaved families throughout the period of loss and loneliness.

Respect for the right of the mentally ill to have the benefit of hospice care at the time of terminal illness is taking shape by way of exploration and planning in a number of hospitals for the mentally ill. Saint Elizabeth's Hospital in Washington, DC, a leader in this movement, has a Hospice Service functioning since October 1979. Here a specially trained team serve as care-givers for the dying patients, in a four- to six-bed unit on a 24-bed intermediate-care ward. The team has a consulting function to all parts of the hospital and serves as a home care team, reaching out to the patients in the family home or foster home. The hospice team is supported by a multidisciplinary staff drawn from other service departments of the hospital. The families of the patients, as well as staff and other patients in the hospital assist in a supporting role, to achieve the underlying objective: 'to provide a better and more appropriate life for terminally ill patients, enabling them to live a life as full and satisfying as possible during their last days, and be free of pain.'

Health Planning Agency guidelines proposed in 1979 indicate the sensitivity to human rights fundamental to the hospice philosophy. The needs of the dying patient for comfort, contact with family and friends, freedom from pain, and reasonable health-care costs, have led to the exploration of alternative approaches to providing care for the terminally ill. Hospice care is the alternative which is currently receiving the greatest scrutiny.

Home care is the focal element and the family and friends of the patient participate actively in the care.

One of the major tenets of most USA hospice programmes is to control pain and other symptoms, but without using artificial means to prolong life. Continuation of medical care is a critical element of hospice services, though the focus is palliative rather than curative.

It is the nature of the services and the underlying philosophy, not the setting, which distinguish a hospice programme from other approaches to terminal care.

Reference

Hammarskjold, Dag. (1964). *Markings*. Translated from the Swedish. Alfred Knopf, New York.

Asia

L. J. de Souza

In the heart of Bombay there looms a great institution which renders yeoman service to the causes of cancer—the Tata Memorial Centre. This hospital is the oldest and largest cancer centre in India catering to over 20 000 new patients and an equal number of follow-up patients every year. I am truly privileged to be one of its staff surgeons.

As a cancer surgeon, one is often made to feel like a demi-God, especially after a tedious and successful cancer operation when your assistants commend your surgery, you yourself feel the satisfaction of a job well done, and the patient looks into your eyes to say 'you have saved my life'. But the surgeon knows deep in his heart that a large percentage of these will return in the throes of terminal cancer when in his total frustration and inadequacy to offer them anything further he will have to say 'Lord help me and the patient, for I can do no more.' It is truly sad that once it becomes apparent that an illness is terminal, conventional medicine often seems unequipped, untrained and even unwilling to deal with death. And yet there is something more we can do. There is a new kind of satisfaction from helping to transform a patient in severe pain into one pain free and at peace. This has been my initiation into hospice care for the advanced cancer patient.

The problems of advanced cancer are common all over the world. These poor individuals have lost the battle with their disease and often await the end in severe pain, depression and loneliness. But in developing countries the problem is aggravated by several factors which are often not fully understood in the West. Let me illustrate with a true example.

One morning while I was going to my office, I was accosted by a wailing woman. I stopped to find out her problems and learnt that she was one of our patients of advanced breast cancer for whom we could do no more. She was left with a huge fungating ulcer on her chest and a body riddled with painful metastases. Her primary problem was excruciating pain. I took her to my office and gave her all the analgesics I could find. She accepted these most gratefully but on going away added 'Doctor, this is not the only pain I have. I have also the pain of hunger for I have not eaten since yesterday!'

It is bad enough to be old and feeble. But to be old, sick with advanced cancer, and poor and hungry with nobody to care for you is often the height of human suffering.

In a developing country like India, I have often been parried with a very difficult question. When a large part of our population is hovering around the starvation line, why are we caring for the dying instead of trying to feed the hungry? To this my simple answer has been, that to relieve one kind of suffering, we cannot neglect another. Both problems have to be tackled, perhaps one more than the other, but always simultaneously.

The solution to the problem in India could perhaps be threefold. The first and the easiest is to turn your face the other way. After all, it is someone else's pain and someone else's problem! But what if that someone was your near and dear one? If you accept the Fatherhood of God, then you must necessarily accept the Brotherhood of Man. How long are we going to turn our heads away from the problem? Euthanasia would indeed be another simple solution, especially in a developing country with several other problems. In over ten years of close contact with cancer patients, I cannot remember a single patient who asked to be put to sleep, especially if he was relieved of his pain adequately and looked after with love. Nobody wants to die. How then can we kill?

Another big problem that we face is that all our hospitals are overcrowded with patients. It is not morally right to block a bed in a specialized hospital for a prolonged period with an advanced and terminal case, when hundreds of patients are waiting for active treatment. Where then are we to send these patients to suffer their agony? The acceptable and humane alternative is a home or hospice where these individuals can be looked after during 'this unique period in the patient's illness when the long defeat of living can be gradually converted into a positive achievement in dying'. To offer this acceptable solution to the problem in our own country, the Shanti Avedna Ashram Trust has been founded. The main aim of this charitable organization is to provide medical and nursing care to the terminally ill cancer patient and to offer this humanitarian service to all those in need of it, free of cost and irrespective of community, caste or creed.

Shanti Avedna Ashram literally means 'Peace in the absence of pain Hospice'—the first of its kind in India. Its aims are beautifully portrayed in our logo which shows a strong hand grasping a weak hand to symbolize relief of pain and consolidation in this trying period, enveloped in the flame of love and under the roof of the Ashram. Our Ashram is still in the planning stage. We hope that it will be functional by next year. Planning is probably the most important stage and I am told that St Christopher's Hospice was planned for several years to make it the fine institution that it is today.

The first and, I thought, major need was to get someone to look after these patients with love. This type of work needs a lot of devotion and cannot be done effectively by poorly paid employees. It is for this reason that I waited till I could get a religious order of Sisters to undertake this work of love. We are lucky to have the sisters of the Holy Cross, an order of trained nurses and hence ideally suited for this task.

The next point was funds. We have been offered help from charitable organizations abroad for the building and equipment. One main worry was how to run it, as it is going to charge no fees and we are not getting any aid from the Government. It was therefore necessary to build a substantial Corpus Fund, which on investment would give us an assured annual income to run the Home. Once people have understood the cause, they are always willing to put in their mite.

We intend to start with only twenty beds. These can be filled up within a few hours considering our acute need. Hence we initially planned to extend it slowly up to 100 beds. I was advised strongly against this by an experienced senior colleague who told me that too much of anything is bad, and with 100 beds the aura of constant suffering and death would be overwhelming. I remembered at this stage a comment made to me by one of the doctors at St Christopher's who said that they had a visiting psychiatrist for the hospice, but perhaps he came more for the benefit of the staff than the patients! Therefore, we have decided to expand to 50 beds only and to start other homes elsewhere as feasible. In fact, our aim is to make the hospice a model we hope many others will follow.

I have incorporated a few points I liked very much at St Christopher's. One is the four-bedded room. It is important not to leave these patients alone. Another feature that I liked was a suitably decorated room adjoining the mortuary where the relations could spend some time with their beloved deceased without disturbing the other patients who themselves are terminal. A further feature which I thought most useful is attaching a blank paper in the patient's chart on which visitors and staff could comment on what the patients said to them. This communication would indeed help in better management. At our centre there will be many patients coming from out of town. We felt it was necessary to have some accommodation for their relations so that they could be close to their dear ones in this trying period and also help with their nursing. We have therefore made provision for this in our plans.

One feature in a home like this is to be strongly stressed. It would be a most convenient place for the unwanted and old and sick to be dumped by their relatives even if they are not terminal cases. At this home, we will of course not be giving active therapeutic treatment. It would be wrong therefore to have any patients there who could benefit from active treatment. To guard against this, especially if influence or pressure is brought to bear, we have a clause in our constitution that requires all patients to be screened by an expert committee of the cancer hospital and considered to be terminal before being admitted to the Ashram.

The mainstay of the Ashram will be of course to make the patient free of pain and the fear of pain. The goal is 'not constant pain but constant relief of pain'. To achieve this we have a specialist volunteer team of a surgeon, two anaesthetists, a neurosurgeon, a psychologist and a rehabilitation therapist who will work in unison. We also plan to have a small theatre for neurosurgical procedures, aspirations, stomas, etc.

Other hospice care in India

There are a few homes for the aged looked after by religious orders scattered over India. There are also very few rehabilitation centres which have a few beds for hospice care. These beds are most certainly grossly inadequate for the acute need of hospice care in our country.

The work of Mother Teresa and her devoted band of sisters has of course made a tremendous inroad towards hospice care in India. To me, Mother Teresa is a living saint and an inspiration. When I went to see her last during her visit to Bombay, I told her that I had to talk on Hospice Care at an International Conference in London and I said I could just not complete my talk without including her work in this field. To this she turned around to me with her sparkling light eyes, smiled and said 'Doctor, it is the Lord's work, not my work'. and went on to add something which she has asked me always to remember—'The moment it becomes your work, everything is lost!' She then told me that she had 98 homes in India looking after the destitute and dying and almost 60 more all over the world. The potent analgesic she uses in all these homes is simply caring for them with 'Love' and perhaps it is so, for in the words of St Augustine 'Where there is love, there is no pain, and if there is pain, it is a pain that is loved.'

However, in order to make 'Love' *the* most potent analgesic we feel it has to be combined with the scientific measures and methods available to us and this is our aim at Shanti Avedna Ashram.

Hospice work in other parts of Asia

It has been very difficult to collect information on hospice work in other parts of Asia, perhaps because so very little of it is being done, as compared to the need for it. We understand that there are some centres in Japan and Singapore offering this service.

In Penang, Malaysia, Mount Miriam Hospital looks after the treatment of terminal cancer patients. It is run by a multiracial community of Franciscan Sisters of the Divine Motherhood. The sisters are highly qualified. Each member of the Order, besides her religious training and formation, acquires a specific expertise in a subject relating to the field of the apostolate in which she labours. Incidentally, it all began in 1967 when Bishop Francis Chan lay dying of cancer and was looked after during his illness by a devoted band of nuns. During this period, he thought of hundreds of others in the same suffering who would never have the love and care given to him. From this came the seeds of 'Mount Miriam' which stands today. I thank God that each one of us does not have to undergo the trials of terminal cancer in order to understand the needs of others. It is enough if we only learn from them.

The task of hospice care in a developing country like India is indeed great and the labourers are few. And yet, as the poet puts it
'The gloom of the world is but a shadow.
Behind it, yet within reach, is joy.
There is radiance and glory in the darkness
Could we but see, and to see
We have to look. I beseech you to look.'
If we have looked at the enormous problem in India and in Asia, there is no doubt we will see and understand it. Thereafter it is up to us to do something about it.

Australia: present and future

Rosemary Howarth

In 1977 the Royal Perth Hospital played host to many hundreds of nurses, doctors, social workers and chaplains from all parts of Australia and New Zealand for two weeks during September. The occasion was the annual postgraduate fortnight organized by the medical and nursing staff, and the theme was 'Cancer'.

The line-up of guest speakers was impressive:

Professor Albert Sabin from USA;

Dr Cicely Saunders from Britain;

Sister Brigid Hirschfield, Grief Counsellor, Queensland;

Douglas Warr, Pharmacist from New Zealand; and

Professor Geoffrey Falkson, Pretoria, South Africa,

and there were many contributions from local doctors, both in hospital practice and in general practice, and from nurses working at the bedside in hospital and the community.

Apart from the packed programme of events in the lecture halls of the hospital for the benefit of staffs of all metropolitan hospitals, there was also a public meeting at the University attended by the Governor of Western Australia and his wife, and as many of the members of the public as could gain access. The hall was packed, with standing room only. Judging from subsequent correspondence received from delegates and members of the public, there was no doubt that the area of greatest interest and concern was that of the needs of the dying patient and his family.

The Australian Hospital Year Book for 1978/79 lists as special areas for the care of the dying:

Caritas Christi Hospice—Kew, Victoria;

Sacred Heart Hospice—Darlinghurst, NSW;

Calvary Hospital—Kogarah, NSW;

Good Shepherd Hospice—Townsville, Queensland.

More recently, the town of Fitzroy, Victoria has allocated eleven beds in a nursing home for hospice care of dying patients. Unfortunately, there have been monumental problems with funding in the case of Fitzroy. Money has not been forthcoming from the Government, so the project was launched with money from public donations with a plan to function on a three-year trial basis. One hopes that at the end of this time there will be some help from State government funds.

On the other side of the map in Western Australia there are no recognized facilities for the care of dying patients and their families, although there are a number of individuals who work quietly in various institutions providing outstanding care for patients and families with the very limited resources available to them. A good example of this is the short-term prognosis area at Mount Henry Hospital in Perth. Situated on a prime site overlooking the Swan River, the hospital incorporates a restorative unit and a unit for permanent care for the aged as part of the Extended Care Service for Perth. A number of beds have been set aside to allow for the admission of patients with a short-term prognosis. The patients go mainly from the oncology units of the metropolitan hospitals for terminal care. The family is very much part of the caring team and are cared for in turn by the staff.

Western Australia comprises one-third of the total area of Australia, although only one-twelfth of the population live here. We take our patients from an area of 11 million square miles from a population of less than 1¼ million people—800 000 of them live in the major urban area of the city of Perth. The problem of distance often necessitates an in-patient stay for people receiving radiotherapy or chemotherapy. The difficulties with family visiting and the expense involved can well be imagined.

During 1979 a small, pleasant area was allocated to the Medical Oncology Service by the ladies of the Red Cross Auxiliary. In these days when the costs of health care delivery are so very high it is doubtful if we could provide many of the services which mean so much to our patients and families if it were not for the superb voluntary services attached to the hospital.

Several minibuses have been donated to the Royal Perth Hospital and with them the services of volunteer drivers who bring our patients from the more distant suburbs of Perth, and in 1979 this splendid group of people financed the transformation from the sow's ear of an old lecture hall to the silk purse of the present Medical Oncology Day Centre to the tune of $35 000.

The Centre was designed to cater for out-patients and day patients receiving chemotherapy. There are only four cubicles but they must be among the most overworked cubicles in the hospital. The area housing the cubicles is bright and cheerful, blue, gold and green being the major colours, carpeted, with piped music, lots of pictures, pot plants, and an atmosphere of welcome.

In my position as Sister-in-Charge of the Oncology Service, I have been responsible for the organization of a planned interdisciplinary programme of total patient care.

The 'back-up' team is quite small. We have the services of half a social worker, a dietician, chaplain, community liaison sister who is our link between the hospital and home, and half an occupational therapist. The occupational therapist, apart from her normal duties, is also our link with the O T Department in the Spinal injuries unit at the Royal Perth Rehabilitation Hospital. They offer their services and expertise in making alterations in the patient's home to allow the family to cope more easily. Ramps may be built for wheelchairs, shower recesses altered and fitted with a seat and hand-held hoses. Alterations may be necessary to the lavatory with the modern preference for low-built pedestals. These alterations can either be temporary or permanent according to family wishes. A donation is welcome but the service is free. The team has a planned meeting each week to discuss all aspects of total care for patient and family, although there are many impromptu meetings between myself and the paramedical staff when intervention is required in times of crisis in the family. I have the earliest contact with patient and family because I visit them on the wards as in-patients. The contact is maintained during out-patient visits and so far I have managed home visits.

The four-cubicle Centre mentioned earlier has become many things to many people. It is very much a 'drop-in' centre for people in trouble, whether they be patients, families or staff. It has also been possible to set aside one of the cubicles to allow for a day admission of a patient being cared for at home to give the family a break. The education of a family member in pain and symptom control has been achieved in the same way. The patient and a family member closely involved in their care have spent a day in the Centre receiving instructions in administration of drugs, particularly when pain is present.

The control of pain and other distressing symptoms is not achieved by the use of medication alone. We can call upon the services of an efficient radiotherapy unit and also upon the services of three enthusiastic anaesthetists who pioneered a Pain Clinic which is now three years old. A welcome addition to our team would be a caring psychiatrist. The emotional resources of people involved with patients with advanced malignant disease are often taxed to the limit and to date this much-needed help has not been forthcoming.

Home care for the patient with terminal illness is provided by nurses from the Silver Chain Nursing Association, founded in 1905 and financed by the people of the State who donated silver coins, mainly shillings. The first district nurse began her duties in 1907 and was provided with a bicycle, a bag for essentials and £2.5s.0d. per week. The Association has gone from strength to strength and the nurses work in homes throughout the State. Several liaison nurses are based in the major teaching hospitals of the State and they form the link between the hospital and the district nurse working in the home. The Association also provides 'extras' such as home help and the loan of aids—wheelchairs, commodes, ripple beds etc.

The link between the Oncology Service and the Cancer Council of West Australia is strong. Thanks to the generosity of the Council, many of our patients are spared the worry of financial hardship, transport costs and the expense of accommodation for a family member in Perth when their home is many hundreds of miles from the city. The Council also provides qualified nursing help in homes to assist the family when death is imminent.

Due to the enormous distances many of our patients travel both for active and for palliative treatment, it is obviously desirable that their last days are spent at home or in any one of thirty-nine small hospitals throughout the State under the care of a GP. The staff of the Oncology Service are 'on call' for advice at all times, but we feel that there is a major task of education to be done in many of these areas.

In January of 1980 the Anglican Archbishop of Perth announced the intention of the Anglican Church to establish a hospice in Perth. The plans are for forty beds, with a religious but non-denominational, medical, non-profit making foundation, supported from the community. We are very excited by the news; we feel this is a major breakthrough.

In the meantime, we shall continue our work in this large teaching hospital experiencing success and failure, frustration and triumph, but caring, sharing and learning always.

Canada: hospice care in Canada

John F. Scott

The past decade

'We stand at a crossroads. The medical and emotional needs of the terminally ill and their families have been defined. The answers are in. It is up to us to determine how long the lag period will be from the accruing of this information to the time when society reaps the benefit.'
(Mount, 1973).

In the early years of the last decade, the pioneers of hospice care in Canada began to ask the right questions. North American literature was focused on the psychological aspects of death and dying. Yet the 1973 study at the Royal Victoria Hospital, Montreal, revealed how often the physical and social problems of patients went unrecognized. In a search for a wholistic solution, Canada discovered the British hospice. In 1970 very few Canadians had ever encountered the word 'hospice'. Yet by the end of the decade, examples of this type of care were enjoying a high reputation. The lay media showed great interest, producing an excellent National Film Board feature film, several videotapes for television and many newspaper and magazine articles. Even more significant, palliative (or hospice) care was a topic of interest in medical journals and at professional conferences. Government health care planners were beginning to evaluate models of hospice care.

While hospice care in the USA grew from home care teams in the direction of autonomous free-standing hospices, the Canadian scene has developed very differently. The Canadian pioneers were committed to the university teaching hospital and it has been in this setting that most developments have occurred. We have attempted to adapt the hospice model of the UK so that it fits within the structure of an active treatment hospital.

Palliative care unit model

Throughout Canada, 'palliative' is the commonly used term for hospice care. Originally employed in Montreal to avoid any francophone misunderstanding of the word 'hospice', palliative also betrays the hospital bias of terminal care in Canada. The palliative care unit (PCU) is being accepted as a special care unit within the acute care hospital with the same geographical and staffing autonomy required by an intensive care unit (ICU) or coronary care unit (CCU). This particular model of terminal care has created unique problems and opportunities. Along with strong physician leadership, this way of organizing terminal care has led to close links between palliative care and active oncology, ensuring constant interaction between 'the care system' and 'the cure system'.

Royal Victoria Hospital, Montreal
Opened in January 1975, this thirteen-bed Unit is a converted ward of the Surgical Pavilion of a university teaching hospital with 800 beds. The Director is Dr B. M. Mount, a urological oncologist. There are two other physicians. Six to 6½ nursing care hours are given per patient per day. The Unit contains advanced cancer patients whose average length of stay is fifteen to twenty days. There is a home care programme run by four PCU-based nurses giving 24-hour coverage.

There is an out-patient clinic and a consultation team for other in-patients who are not suitable for (or are awaiting) transfer. Support services to the patients' families and bereavement follow-up are supplied. With a strong emphasis on education and research, this centre has become the teaching model for terminal care in Canada.

St Boniface Hospital, Winnipeg
This hospital is affiliated with the University of Manitoba. In late 1974, a 22-bed Terminal Care Unit was opened in the geriatric wing of the hospital. The full-time Director is Dr Paul Henteleff. The length of stay of the patients is about twenty-one days. The Home Care Co-ordinator follows the progress of sixty patients and nursing care is provided by community visiting nurses.

Salvation Army Grace Hospital, Toronto
This is a 110-bed chronic care hospital in central Toronto, close to the Princess Margaret Hospital, the largest cancer treatment centre in Ontario. In January, 1979, a fifteen-bed Palliative Care Unit was opened on the top floor of the hospital and this is funded by the provincial Ministry of Health. The Director is Dr Margaret Scott. Nursing is at 'hospice' levels (in Canada this is approximately six to seven nursing hours per patient per day before vacation and sick days are considered).

Hôpital Notre-Dame, Montréal
This 800-bed teaching hospital of L'Université de Montréal opened a twelve-bed Unité de soins palliatifs in May 1979 in a renovated ward.

Home care is carried out by L'Association de l'Entraide Ville-Marie (AEV) and there is a separate visiting nurse service for terminally ill patients. The AEV cares for francophone patients from any Université de Montréal hospital.

St Clare Mercy Hospital, St John's, Newfoundland
In November 1979, this 325-bed teaching hospital of Memorial University opened a ten-bed Palliative Care Unit. The province supplies 80 per cent of its funding and 20 per cent comes from religious orders and private sources. There is one part-time physician and ten beds are available for families when needed.

Some chronic care institutions in Canada, which have traditionally cared for dying patients with advanced cancer, have attempted gradually to upgrade and co-ordinate their care and educate their staff. For example, Riverdale Hospital, Toronto has centralized terminal care on a forty-bed ward. Through the efforts of Dr Montague, they are gradually increasing the nursing levels and paramedical support services.

Consultation team model

Several centres in Ontario have attempted to improve the quality of terminal care in their hospitals by developing a Palliative Care Consultation Service. In this model of care an interdisciplinary team assesses all terminally ill patients, gives advice on symptom control and provides continuing support to patients, families and staff.

The type of service offered varies greatly from one centre to another. Some begin as a committee of professionals, all with full-time positions in other fields. They offer advice to hospital staff on terminal care for a few hours per week. Some teams are led by a nurse or social worker with little or no physician involvement. Some teams concentrate on in-service education and psychosocial aspects of care.

When political or economic factors rule out a palliative care unit or free-standing hospice, or when a community hospital has too small a cancer population to justify a unit, the symptom control team is an efficient way of improving care. While the nurse may co-ordinate the team's activities, there must be strong leadership from a physician who is available for consultations throughout the week.

The experience at St Michael's Hospital has shown how marked an impact such a team can have on care, yet the scope of this model is limited. There is insufficient control over the environment, medical decisions and staff selection. The care provided over the twenty-four hours is inconsistent and unco-ordinated. This model does not solve one of the basic problems—the lack of nursing care available at the bedside.

The next decade

In April 1980, the first free-standing hospice in Canada opened in Quebec City, funded by the provincial branch of the Canadian Cancer Society. Although autonomous, La Maison de Sillery is directed by a medical oncologist, Dr Louis Dionne, and is closely affiliated to L'Hôtel-Dieu de Quebec, a teaching hospital of Laval University.

At least three other centres hope to open palliative care units in the next year:

St Michael's Hospital, Toronto;
Vancouver General Hospital, Vancouver;
University of Western Ontario, London.

There are several other hospitals (Victoria, Calgary, Edmonton, Hamilton, Windsor) who are actively investigating feasibility and funding for a unit.

The consultation team model will also continue to spread and influence care. New teams are being established at:

McMaster Medical Centre, Hamilton, Ontario;
Mississauga General, Mississauga, Ontario;
Oakville Trafalgar Hospital, Oakville, Ontario;
Metropolitan Hospital, Windsor, Ontario.

We must encourage strong physician involvement. While emotional, spiritual and family support services are essential, symptom control must be the first priority of palliative care. The presence of such a team teaching and assisting staff will undoubtedly have a positive influence on the care provided to all patients—acute, chronic and terminal—since many of the principles of hospice care are adaptable to health care generally.

Government planning

The Department of National Health and Welfare has recently formed a working group to establish guidelines on the development of palliative care in Canada. This small committee includes the medical directors of three palliative care units (RVH, Montreal; Winnipeg; and Grace, Toronto) to ensure that these guidelines are both clinically sound and follow in the hospice tradition.

While this national group will have a powerful influence on development, the actual delivery of health care in Canada is a provincial responsibility. The Ministries of Health in Quebec, Manitoba, Ontario, Alberta, British Columbia and Newfoundland have all been actively involved in evaluating the hospice concept. In British Columbia, for example, the recent government study has led to their decision to open two palliative care units, one in each of the two major cities, Victoria and Vancouver.

Regional co-ordination

The six teaching hospitals of McGill University, Montreal, have approved a plan to provide comprehensive and co-ordinated care to all their in-patients and out-patients who require palliative care. A central hospice or palliative care unit will be established on the island of Montreal and will admit patients from all McGill hospitals. Each participating hospital would set up a consultation symptom-control team. The PCU at the Royal Victoria Hospital would be one component of this larger plan. Other hospitals with large cancer populations might also choose to set up a small PCU as well as a consultation team. A city-wide home care programme based at the central PCU would offer home care to patients from all McGill hospitals. A similar regional home care programme is planned for Calgary.

University education

A Chair in Palliative Care has been endowed at the Faculty of Medicine, University of Western Ontario, London, Ontario. The University is presently accepting applications, hoping such a position will attract an experienced physician who will establish and direct a PCU in a university hospital as well as institute an education programme for students of medicine and other health care disciplines (at basic science, clinical and postgraduate levels).

This is the most concrete example of a growing interest to integrate hospice care into the university education of physicians and nurses. Medical educators are beginning to recognize the need to improve the teaching of symptom control. They also realize the potential of the hospice concept to 'humanize' all of health care.

Research

The National Cancer Institute of Canada, the major funding body for cancer research, has recently decided to stimulate research into the quality of life for cancer patients. They have made palliative care their special interest and already over forty research applications are under study. The first of several national workshops was held in Toronto in April 1980 to study these proposed projects and stimulate further research in the field of palliative care.

Facing unique difficulties and possessing unique resources, each community and nation represented at this Conference will find diverse ways of meeting the challenge of hospice care. Yet we are united by our patients who issue to all of us the same urgent demand for better care and the same gentle invitation to watch with them.

Reference

Mount, Balfour M. (1973–4) Death—a Part of Life? *Crux* **II**, No. 3. p.7.

Netherlands: development of terminal care in the Netherlands

Marlijn de Jong-Vekemans

The translation of Dr E. Kubler Ross's book, *On Death and Dying*, was initially responsible for the change in approach in the Netherlands to the seriously sick person who was expected to die within a short period.

In 1969 small groups of general practitioners who had read the book discussed it with each other and began examining the possibilities within their own practices of how to use it. In addition, a small group of nurses, nursing aides, chaplains and psychologists began increasingly to question what was being done in this specific field of health care.

In 1972—during my training at a high school for nurses—I had the opportunity of meeting Professor Dr L. J. Menges, clinical psychologist. In his lectures he expressed a vision and sensitivity for the care and attention in that difficult phase of a patient's sickness when it becomes clear there is no more chance of recuperation. After I finished my studies I was able to take part in a work group under his leadership in Leiden. In 1973 this group began to study published material on this subject and to discuss jointly our approach and care for the seriously ill person. This work group consisted of: a psychologist, 2 chaplains, 2 doctors, 3 nurses and a nursing aide. The purpose of this group was focused on eventually forming special units for terminal patients within the existing nursing homes (every Dutch nursing home has terminal patients besides the other two categories—chronically sick and rehabilitation patients). The question arose *how* we fulfil, for the terminally ill, the traditional nursing home function of care and counselling to the end, preferably in direct co-operation with the family.

Besides this work group a special committee was formed, the members of which consisted of a professor in radiology, two specialists of internal medicine and a directrice of a general large hospital. The purpose of this committee was to support us and more especially to meet with the Ministry of Health with the purpose of getting Government subsidy for this specific field. Both the work group and the special committee were in agreement that the employment of extra staff to assure continuity and the availability of proper facilities were primary necessities.

During these two years many letters were written to the Minister of Health and several meetings took place to discuss this project. However, at the end of 1974 there was an unexpected but definite announcement from the Government of a decrease of employment in the health care field. An attempt was then made via one of the Church Foundations in Holland (Diaconessen) to receive subsidy, and several private foundations were written to. Unfortunately, both efforts were unsuccessful.

By 1975 the work group had the impression that all their work had been done for nothing. But then contact was made with Dr T. West of St Christopher's Hospice, who was attending a Congress of Terminal Care in Holland. Professor L. J. Menges had a talk with him and discussed our problems. It was suggested that one of the members of the work group could be sent to London for study and practical experience. From publications we all knew that Dr Cicely Saunders' hospice only came about because of tremendous effort, sacrifice, patience and a never wavering courage. In March 1975 I went for the first time to St Christopher's Hospice. In the meantime, a very good documentary appeared on the Dutch television about Cicely Saunders and St Christopher's and this programme influenced public opinion. Many people began to say 'When my time comes, I should like to die in a place like St Christopher's.' Fortunately, the reaction to the programme was not a passing emotion, but in several places in Holland particular initiatives were taken. For example, training centres in health care started to ask for information from the few who had practical experience. After my visit and work in St Christopher's, I myself spoke in nurses' training schools, with social workers, nursing aides, volunteer groups, doctors and medical students and had discussions about the world and the care of the seriously sick. Over time more and more requests arrived from those who were looking for a better approach to the counselling of the dying.

In spite of these encouraging developments, there was still scepticism about the counselling of terminal patients and their families. Large general hospitals—and especially Government agencies—kept to their standpoint that this counselling should be done by the patient's family and that institutions should not be established for the dying. The Government saw the counselling of the dying as 'dangerous'. Experiments might be carried out with the dying person. The gap between those working with the dying and those on whom decisions about subsidizing this specific help rested seemed to be growing wider and wider.

At the end of 1976, the Minister of Health and Environment held preparatory talks in order to set up the Project Group Terminal Care, the function of which would be to decide on the desirability of a project on counselling of the dying, to formulate the purpose of such a project and research the possibilities for the establishment. The Group met six times and presented a report to the Secretary of Health in November, 1977. Meanwhile, in August 1977, after a long period of preparation, a project was started in the Antonius Ijsselmonde Nursing Home in Rotterdam, funded by the City. With the available funds, only one full-time psychologist and a part-time nurse (who was specially trained in this field) could be employed. It was thought by some that Antonius Ijsselmonde would be a terminal home comparable to St Christopher's in London, but this has never been the intention. Time will have to make clear if a special department or unit for terminal patients should be created. For the present the purpose is to try to fit the project into the existing structure of the nursing home and to evaluate the result. This experience will be the subject of a report and the knowledge acquired will be available to everyone involved in providing help to the seriously ill.

In April, 1979 we received official notice from the Government that we would receive subsidy for the project Terminal Care. Although there is much justified joy in getting this subsidy, we realize very well that a new responsibility has been put on our shoulders. We see our task as setting an example for all nursing homes in Holland so that further positive improvements will lead to more and better care for all terminal patients.

Sweden: the impact of hospice care in Sweden

Loma Feigenberg

The hospice and its influence on Sweden can be seen from at least two viewpoints. First, in terms of the number of real institutions which are functioning or at least are planned. Second, as regards the impact of the hospice movement on care of the dying generally.

The first aspect can be dealt with quite briefly. In Sweden it is often said that innovations from abroad take a decade to catch on. Somewhat more than ten years have now passed for the hospice movement and the first signs of real activity in terms of hospice-like units are in fact starting to appear. In Stockholm the only existing religiously oriented hospital is planning a unit, not in the hospital itself but in an adjacent building, which will be devoted to the care of dying patients. The start is expected in about two years' time. In the south of Sweden, in the town of Halmstad, Dr Lars Risholm is beginning to plan for a similar unit. Ulla Qvarnstrom, a nurse who left Sweden recently, has been involved in the planning of hospices. Some projects are beginning to take shape in Goteborg. All this means that no hospices are functioning yet in Sweden but plans are under way in some places.

Turning instead to the impact of the hospice movement on care of the dying, the effects are much more extensive. In Sweden, as everywhere, awareness of problems of death and dying has been influenced greatly by experience from St Christopher's Hospice. Nurses, doctors and hospital administrators have started to think, discuss and publish materials inspired by the hospice movement. As much as five years ago a Government Sub-committee was appointed with the aim of looking into 'questions relating to medical care in the terminal phase of life'. In the Committee report, which appeared recently, it is above all the emphasis on policy for the treatment of pain which has been profoundly influenced by experience at St Christopher's.

In this context it is necessary to note that medical administration and social organization differ somewhat in Great Britain and Sweden. Our committee has stated that hospices are important and influential institutions. Experience from them must be used and extended. But we do not propose that the Government should actively stimulate the setting-up of hospices. We are not against the idea of building hospices or similar units in Sweden on an experimental basis, so that results in other countries can be compared with what can be achieved in our country. Such units can also serve an educational purpose. But what the report chiefly stresses is the need to teach everybody on every level in the medical system to increase both their awareness of the problems and their ability to give appropriate psychological care to dying people. In assessing this approach it should be remembered that Sweden has a small population which is accustomed to rather uniform medical care. Moreover, this care does not place a financial burden on the patient. It is planned from an administrative centre and evolves along the same lines all over the country, though it is actually provided by local authorities.

As for the future, so many other issues involving death and dying dominate our anxieties and fantasies today that it is becoming increasingly difficult to sort them out. Death is so prominent that it is difficult to forecast the development of terminal care in the sense in which we use this term here today. We have the feeling even in the medical profession that death is being taken out of our hands, we are losing control and deep down we are growing anxious. But if we nevertheless try to focus on what we look upon as our professional work or obligation, it is my feeling that the effort in Sweden will be to start some courses, give more lectures, and train all groups of medical professionals so that they are better able to care for dying patients. In other words, death education will reach as many of those in health care as ever possible. This goal will take more time but it will also reach more people than if we started hospices with a staff trained for that kind of work. Roughly 85 000 human beings die each year in Sweden (1 per cent of the population). Even if we deduct those who can and want to die at home, as well as those who die in the street, there would still not be the resources or the manpower to let the rest benefit from hospice care. We also feel that to take away the dying from existing institutions would be detrimental for the psychological atmosphere of medical care in general. It is, on the contrary, important to stress and acknowledge the actuality and nearness of death and the danger of dying in every health care setting. My impression is, therefore, that in Sweden energy will be devoted to more general, long-term planning for care of the dying, involving all those engaged in our country's medical system. This will be a development along the lines of the social structures that have existed for decades. From the hospice movement it will probably take over more of the humane approach, the fight against pain and the concern for the family than of the actual organizational setting.

Great Britain: the hospice in Britain

Eric Wilkes

There are now fifty to sixty operational units dedicated to some kind of service to the dying patient and the family. Many more units are at the planning stage but most of these are not likely, without major shifts in design, to get beyond that stage. What, in this busy decade of industry and devotion and change, have we to show for our efforts?

First, the growth of the hospice concept demonstrates the dissatisfaction with, and the inadequacy of, a rather depersonalized system of medicine, for all the tremendous number of gratifying and impressive exceptions proving this rule. Because of our work, the care of the dying patient, the support of the relatives, the training of doctors, nurses and rehabilitation professionals, will never be quite the same again. But now we come to a less popular and a less easily acceptable argument. We have shared in some of the errors and misconceptions of our own health care system. Whether we have a small unit of very few beds in the community, a sixty- or seventy-bed unit like St Christopher's or, commonest of all, a 25-bed unit (as about the smallest economically viable unit), we have shared the prevailing and improper preoccupation with beds. The National Health Service has spent millions of pounds on buildings and beds when we should have spent less on replacing our shabby, out-dated buildings and more on services and pairs of hands.

It is time to pray that the American hospice movement will not be so fashionable and powerful that they in turn will be corrupted by plentiful and indiscriminate funding to be spent on buildings just at the time when the British hospice movement has so much to learn from them. Over-bedded though many American cities are, we British have with difficulty created beds which stand empty for lack of funding. We do not wish to persevere in policies that are being overtaken by events, with our well-designed wards too lying empty for lack of funds. In the future every brick we place on top of another brick to help a dying patient will need to be costed against the benefits that money could have funded in terms of community nursing services. In Sheffield, where I work, we are expecting 29 per cent more patients over the age of 75 by 1986 than we have now. Fifteen per cent of cases dying of cancer at home are cared for by relatives themselves over 70 years of age. Most patients die in hospital, yet most of those dying in the acute wards have spent most of their last month of life at home. The final admission lasts, for the majority, less than two weeks. A quarter of our admissions to St Luke's are dead in three days. The commonest single reason for admission to St Luke's is to give respite to an exhausted or frightened family. Some beds will be necessary—indeed vital—but we must be in the forefront of the battle to improve the simple community services that could up-grade home care and reduce the need for many of these expensive beds.

Terminal care units should be of the highest quality or should not be called into existence at all. Yet inflation cannot be waved away. The Sheffield Unit that cost £120 000 eight years ago now has an insurance value of over £1 million. Our annual budget is well over £300 000. A one-to-one nurse : patient ratio may be essential to deal with the difficult cases that properly should come to us, yet recent salary increases to nurses, however inadequate or justified or overdue, are not easily funded. Nurses' salaries are the biggest single item of the NHS budget, and to attract money for what is likely to be in essence an additional nursing unit such as a new hospice, there must be something very special to offer to gain the necessary support. Such support nowadays is to be classed as perfectly possible but unlikely. The herding together of those soon to die is an unattractive concept, justified only because in fact it works surprisingly well. It is still possibly thought of as an affront, however unintentional, to doctors and nurses who are doing their best, and their naturally cautious reaction will at times move over into a frank hostility heightened in America by the potential loss of fees.

Therefore, difficult relationships with our colleagues in the traditional apparatus of care are to be expected, and neither are hospice personnel themselves saintly and without blemish. It is possible that the independent and physically separate charities lead to an isolation that tempts towards arrogance or complacency, a feeling that 'only hospice units do it properly'.

In fact, only some 10 per cent of local cancer deaths occur in the special Unit in Sheffield and the national average must be less than half that figure. The NHS continuing-care units built clost to or as part of a NHS hospital are also not without their disadvantages. They can be victimized by an impoverished administration and, by their very situation, deprived of imagination and resources. It is not likely that the Sheffield Unit could have recruited anything like our 300 volunteers if we were sited in an ordinary district general hospital. There is no clear reason to strangers why our hospice amenities should be maintained at a higher level than anyone else's, unless we are—as we should be—classed as a rather special kind of intensive care.

Our problems do not end here. The commonest admissions to hospice units are primary tumours of lung and breast. The national use of tobacco is probably past its peak and if we could find any effective treatment for breast cancer—other than the preventive measure of breeding young—then the hospice beds of today would be half-empty and of doubtful viability. We must plan for our own obsolescence whilst providing counselling, support and good symptom-control for patients and relatives, a base for a vast change in attitudes amongst our professional colleagues, an up-grading of community terminal care, including day-care, and a vigorous teaching programme especially centred on the needs of young doctors and nurses in training. This programme makes special centres associated with schools of medicine and nursing justifiable. We see, therefore, tomorrow's hospice as having a few beds, but not necessarily in a special unit on its own; as a nursing support service that bulldozes away the administrative tank-traps that separate hospital and community; and a competent deprofessionalization of care led by professionals exceptionally competent in their field, who will carry the hospice approach, without more vulgarization than is implicit in such a leadership role, throughout the health service.

8
Achievement, failure and the future: hospice analysed

Paul Torrens

When I began to be interested in hospice work, four or five years ago, like everyone else I immediately became aware of the pre-eminence of Dr Cicely Saunders and the group at St Christopher's and I must also admit that I immediately developed a sense of unease about Dr Saunders without having ever met her. It seemed to me that everything that I had read and heard about her and her work indicated so effective, so wise, so compassionate an approach towards the well-being of dying human beings, that it simply could not be true.

I have had many experiences in my life of meeting and working with 'famous people', most of whom, on closer association, became less God-like and more like the rest of us. And indeed, I found, as I came in contact with some of them, that not only were they idols with feet of clay, but in at least one case the clay had infiltrated upward through the body and was now residing almost solely in the brain. For that reason I was really rather apprehensive about ever meeting or working with Dr Saunders and her associates in the flesh, since I was sure that no one could be that good and still be alive.

One day, however, I was reading some of Dr Saunders' writings and I came across a chapter that she had done for a textbook in which she said, in effect 'We have reached a place in hospice work where there are now a lot of inbred beliefs that have become sacred cows. If I could think of the most constructive thing that I could do to improve hospice work myself, for the future, I think it would be to conduct a sacred cow shoot, so that the field could go ahead with a new kind of insight and freedom from past practices.' I immediately changed my views about Dr Saunders. I am intrigued with the vision of a sacred cow shoot, and I want to look realistically and honestly at what we have accomplished and what we have learned in the hospice movement, and also at what we have not accomplished and perhaps what we have not learned. I do this, not from the point of view of the cold, abstract or disinterested critic, since I feel that no one who is connected with this kind of work for any length of time, if he is a person of any wit or warmth, can remain disinterested or untouched either by the work or the workers. I plead guilty to being a partisan of the effort to improve the care of dying patients, indeed, the care of all patients. On the other hand, I have been a student of health care systems throughout the world and I think I have developed a broad perspective on the health needs of people in general. I would like to bring that broader view into play and place hospice programmes in the setting of the broader health care systems that serve people all over the world.

First of all, what have we learned and what have we accomplished? It is obvious that we have learned a great deal about death itself, particularly death from cancer. As a result of looking steadily into the eyes of dying patients and their families year in and year out, we now know much more about what it is like to die, what it is like to have a loved one die and what it is like to care for them both. It seems incredible to think that it has only been in the last ten years that we as doctors, nurses and professionals of all kinds have focused our attention to any great degree on the process of dying; that we have begun to devote the kind of intelligent and careful attention to death that we had previously lavished on much less important, but much more scientifically attractive, events.

Second, in learning about death, we have also learned a tremendous amount about how to care for the dying and their loved ones. We have learned what dying patients and their families need, and how to provide these things in a better form, with better grace and with better effect. Learning more about death and dying, we have learned to marshal our strengths, talents and resources to organize better programmes of care, to enlist the wide range of professional, non-professional, lay, volunteer and family energy. At least now we know how to care for the dying, how to make their final days more comfortable and more fulfilling. We know how to do our side of things better, better focus our energies and our programmes.

Third, in the process of learning about death and about caring for the dying, I would venture to say that everyone involved has learned a tremendous amount about him- or her-self. We have been forced and challenged, in a way that never really took place before, to examine ourselves, our values and our behaviours, and our reasons for being what we are and doing whatever it is that we do—in short, to look inward in a way that perhaps might never have been done if we had not been involved in this work. I frankly have yet to meet a person, whether professional or lay, who has worked for any time around dying patients and who has not become much more introspective and fuller of insight about themselves.

Finally, it seems clear that all of us, by looking at and becoming more comfortable with death, both with the deaths of others and the inevitable deaths of ourselves, have begun to learn more about life. We have realized that although this time we are the rowers in the boat across the River Styx and others are passengers, the day will come when we change places and others will row for us as we move on to that place where so many of our patients go now. As with developing more self-awareness, I would also venture to say that I have not met a person working with the dying who has not developed a better sense of living, of life, particularly of his own or her own life and its values, joys and beauties.

What has been accomplished as a result of these learned truths? What can we look back on as a record of achievements during these past ten years of effort? The first has been the development of a model of the better process of dying and, more important, a better programme for the care of the dying. The principles and practices that we in the hospice movement take so much for granted nowadays have taken years of work at St Christopher's, St Joseph's in Hackney, in Dublin and elsewhere. We have had to assemble bit by bit, piece by piece, the basic elements of a good programme of care for the dying. People around the world have had to test, revise and test again many times over, putting together the final outline of the programme we would all recognize as the standard hospice model for the care of the dying. We tend nowadays to presume it always existed. It seems to have happened so easily; it has been so easy to absorb and to agree with. It has not happened easily. It is a major achievement and a significant one.

Second, not only has the basic model been developed, it is now being replicated in programmes all over the world, in a great variety of slightly, sometimes widely, divergent programmes. In the United States alone there have been possibly 250 programmes, of one form or another; in Canada another 25 to 50; in England, Scotland and Wales perhaps an additional 50. Around the world, who knows, there are perhaps an additional 50 to 100. In this short period of time, most probably within the last five years, a network of 400 programmes, institutions or community efforts of one kind or another, have been developed for the care of the dying, trying in some fashion or another to include the elements of the original model of care that has been St Christopher's. In perhaps 400 or more places around the earth professionals are providing better care for dying patients and that unique, blessed kind of care. This is no mean accomplishment and one that Dr Saunders, Dr West and the staff at St Christopher's can well be proud of. The seeds of their work have been sown around the world to grow, thrive and provide care for the dying and their families, and to educate society how to do that work better.

A further achievement that I would wish to be sure credit is taken for is the tremendous amount of education that has taken place among the public and among professionals with regard to death and dying. In my work at UCLA I teach not only in the School of Public Health but in the School of Medicine and the School of Nursing and I am continuously amazed at the interest shown by professional students in the care of the dying and the independent reading that they have done. In my experience around UCLA, it has been very evident that involving students in work with dying patients has been one of the best ways of re-focusing and re-channelling their interests away from the more sterile and abstract pursuit of the laboratories and back to the bedside of the patients themselves; back to working with people; to understanding the aspirations of life and the tragedies of death, in short, to those things that make medical students and nursing students better doctors and better nurses. This has been a remarkable achievement, not to be passed over too easily. It has changed values and, more importantly, it has laid down a broad base of movement upon which changes within professional values and thoughts are even now taking place.

Tied in with this achievement of broader education of both public and professionals, I would point out the significant achievement in programmes of care of the dying that are not in hospices or similar special activities. It seems apparent that the wave of enthusiasm for starting new hospice programmes, in the United States at least, is waning. Preliminary figures that I have looked at recently would suggest that there is not the great energetic development of new programmes all over the country that one saw just two years ago. Instead, there seems a quite different phenomenon taking place—the phenomenon of the standard programmes of care, that is the non-hospice programmes of care, the traditional doctor in hospital and nursing home programmes of care which many of us despaired of for so long. These programmes are now beginning to undergo change and metamorphosis on the basis of what they have seen and learned in hospice systems. On all sides in southern California I see the traditional programmes of care for dying patients in traditional hospitals with traditional doctors, now being expanded and having particular services added to them that were simply not there before—a nurse, a social worker, a counsellor, home care services, transportation or even day hospitals developed where none existed before. None of these programmes calls itself a hospice. Indeed, there are a number of cases in which they are very proud to point out that they are not hospices, simply 'good programmes of care that we've always been doing'. Whether in fact they have always been doing it or not is beside the point! The important thing is that there is a great deal of change going on.

It is very hard to document this latest wave of development. It has taken place quietly and unobtrusively, involving the addition of a single nurse here or a psychiatric consultant there or a small counselling programme somewhere else. It is hard to document these small increments of change, and yet they are all about us. And that may perhaps be the most significant achievement of all: that the development of hospice programmes has brought about quietly and gradually, but significantly, an improvement and upgrading of the programmes of the care for the dying in the standard, traditional or conventional settings where, in fact, most people die.

So much for the good news. Now what have we not learned and not accomplished? First of all, we really have not documented in an exact, clear and well-reported way whether hospice programmes for the care of the dying make a difference. That they make a difference is generally acknowledged. However, when one goes to look for statistics to support this contention, they simply are not there, or at least they are not there in the form that a careful and thoughtful and exacting intelligence would require. When one looks for hard data, well-controlled studies of a more scientific nature, objective measures of outcome on hospice programmes, one finds that the facts are not available. With the exception of a few major studies carried out by people like Robert Twycross, John Hinton, Colin Murray

Parkes, one simply does not find the wealth of objective evidence that really should be there. We have not documented our undoubted achievements very well or, in some cases, at all.

Not only have we not done a very good job of measuring accurately the results of our work, we have also failed to show that the work is that much better than the care of the dying that is given to patients in settings other than formal hospice programmes.

We in the hospice movement know, as an article of faith, that hospice programmes clearly do a better job. We know it because most of us started in the others and despaired of them. Unfortunately, however, that is not really enough. It represents believers saying, 'I have a better religion than you'. It may in fact be true. But just as we have failed to document the results of our work very well, so we have failed to document that the results of that work are that much better than the results of others. We presume it and we believe it, but we have not made it a point to engage ourselves in carefully controlled studies to show how much better hospice work is than the traditional care of the dying. To carry that a step further, I must further point out that we have not documented very well the cost of what we are doing, nor done a very effective job of either pointing out that our services are less expensive than traditional services for example (if that is the case), or where the expenses are more, giving reasons why that is justified. We have not, in brief, carried out the types of critical, even sceptical, cost-benefit analyses that are becoming more and more a part of the health care world.

In a quite different arena, it must be said that we have learned a tremendous amount about the care of the dying, but mostly limited to the care of those dying with cancer, particularly with the care of the dying cancer patient who is dying relatively quickly, or at least within a rather limited time span. We have selected a certain kind of dying patient to work with. We have not learned a great deal about other dying patients; patients who die more slowly, whose movement from life to death is much more gradual, even while it is just as inexorable. We have not come to grips with some of the other chronic disease conditions which lead just as clearly, just as certainly, to death, only in a different time frame. The idea of taking the principles of what we have learned and applying them to a different pattern of death is most important.

In yet another vein, it should be pointed out that we have not really yet learned how to diagnose a community's real need for a hospice programme or for a programme for the care of the terminally ill, nor have we really learned how to plan for the development of organized programmes in communities that do not have any yet. What we have seen is a tremendous amount of spontaneous enthusiasm; the result is that we have programmes in various parts of the USA that were started in the image of their founders, but not in the image of their patients or their community's needs.

At the present time there are 40 organized programmes of care for the terminally ill in the State of California, 20 in southern California alone. Personally, I do not have the faintest idea, nor does anyone that I know, whether we need 20 such programmes or 2 or 200.

Of course, the most important shortfall of all is simply the shortage of finance. Somehow or other we in the hospice movement have not yet been able to get ourselves implanted into the traditional mainstream of health and medical care that would ensure the long-term life of our programmes. There has been an amazing amount of creative work done in the raising of money—including creative book-keeping and accountancy that shifts funds from one part of the hospital to another—but the bloodstream (if one looks at finance as blood, and indeed in organizational life it is) has simply not been well established yet. So our programmes are in danger almost daily of a change of government programme, of policy, or personnel, the withdrawal of a wealthy donor who has provided most of the funds. In short, our programmes are in great jeopardy.

How, then, do we prepare for the future? Taking what we have accomplished on the one hand, and it is so substantial, and what we have not accomplished on the other, how do we put these two together and neither be desperately depressed nor so exhilarated that we ignore things that are important to do?

We must begin to prepare ourselves for some changes in attitude with regard to hospice programmes. We may begin to find that the success of our programmes begins to be captured by others, without any credit to us. The fire that we have nurtured for so many years may very well be stolen away to be 'better used'. We may be left saying, 'but that's our work'. I think it very important that we begin to see that in fact that may be a very good thing and an achievement.

My own prediction is that there will continue to be need for special units for the care of the dying and the terminally ill all around the world. But they will increasingly be, I think, units for teaching, research and the special functions that can only be carried out in them, rather than for the broad service functions that many carry out now. I see those broad service functions being carried out in a much wider range of places. Moreover, for the future the question of financing will become increasingly critical. I feel confident it will be solved by involvement with health insurance plans, the national health services and so on. That will, I think, be very good but it will present certain kinds of problems. For one thing, there will clearly be additional paper work and regulation, and we will increasingly be bound down in other people's directives. We have had the luxury of developing a programme freely, outside of the constraints of much of the organized health care system, to the great benefit of patients. The price we will pay for having better financial support may well be more regulation.

How about us in the hospice movement as individuals? How do we as people go about preparing for the future? I think one thing we all must begin to do for our own future is to be much more analytically critical of ourselves and our work; much more carefully sceptical of our motives and our efforts—and I mean positive scepticism. How many of us, for example, have really looked at our own motives for doing this work? How much of it is really tied up with what we get back from patients that makes us feel good, and how much with what we give them? How much of what we do is tied up in good work because it is new and innovative and creative? As we move into the future, when it no longer becomes quite so new, innovative and creative, how do we deal with that?

In fact, I think we deal with it by returning once again to the direct care of patients. But for many of us it is very important to realize why we are working, so that when the difficult days do come we can say 'I knew this was going to happen and I am in this work because I like what I am able to give to patients'.

In the same vein, we must turn carefully and analytically to examine our programmes, to document their efforts and particularly their effects better. Any programme of caring for the dying that does not make a deliberate and concerted effort to document and measure exactly what is being done and what is being achieved should be seen as lacking in that critical ingredient of self-review and appraisal and therefore as seriously deficient. It may well be that when we start to do this, we find that our work is really not so good in one area as we thought, and much better in another. We may find our communities need things that are quite different from what we thought, and indeed that what we are doing in one area might be exactly what they do need. In short, our progress through the future should be based more on fact than on assumption, presumption or traditional beliefs.

Finally, I would say that we must come to grips with a fundamental reality if we are to move into the future strongly. That reality is that in the future we are going to have to make peace, in the first instance with the traditional medical, nursing and hospital establishment and in the second instance with bureaucrats, economists, social planners and all that ilk. We have, on some occasions, done a very effective job of wounding our colleagues to the extent that they do not like to deal with us in some very important ways. We may have done it without knowing it, without intent, but I would have to say that in many ways our colleagues look at us as morally prissy people who believe we are always in the right and they are always in the wrong. But our future is tied up with our colleagues and somehow or other we will have to come to terms with the fact that they are as good as us in many ways—as kind as us, as busy as us, maybe not as insightful as us, but our colleagues, nevertheless, with whom we must work.

The same holds true of the administrators, and I would point specifically to the economists who now begin to influence and control so much of the flow of money. Economic theory and cost-effect analysis—these are the laser beam weapons of the future that these people wield with such skill (I think it is skill). In our modern society, it is the economists and administrators who very often are able either to channel resources to good work or keep it from coming. Those of us who have said bureaucracy is a perjorative word must begin to think very seriously about that, and I think honestly to realize that administrators are people, albeit going about different purposes differently. There is no way that the principles that have been so carefully nurtured at St Christopher's and other places around the world can go ahead without the support of the economists and the political bureaucracy in which we exist.

Challenge for the future, then, lies no longer in the traditional areas—the simple struggle for existence and identity. That challenge has been met and largely overcome. The challenge now is to refine, to reappraise; to evaluate that identity and the separate parts of it that make up our various programmes; to match that identity and its parts better to the needs of our communities and our cultures; to try new approaches and new linkages; to move into new areas, so that the work we have started well will serve as a leaven and as a catalyst for future developments.

These will be very trying days ahead of us, perhaps more confusing and trying than the original days. Early on it was clear who the villains and the heroes were, where the challenges lay, what were the pitfalls to be avoided. There was the good work and it was easy to devote one's life, twenty-four hours a day, to that work because it was quite clear. I think now we have passed that stage and ahead lie many diverse paths, many confusions of a subtler nature. It will take exactly the same strength, vigour, education, insight and dedication that the work at St Christopher's, starting thirteen years ago, demanded.

Index